MW01078254

PEARLS & PITFALLS IN ELECTROCARDIOGRAPHY

PITHY, PRACTICAL POINTERS

Second Edition

PEARLS & PITFALLS IN ELECTROCARDIOGRAPHY

PITHY, PRACTICAL POINTERS

Second Edition

HENRY J. L. MARRIOTT, M.D., F.A.C.P, F.A.C.C.

Director, Shick Cardiac Education Center
Naples Community Hospital
Naples, Florida
Clinical Professor of Medicine (Cardiology)
Emory University, Atlanta, Georgia
Clinical Professor of Pediatrics (Cardiology)
University of Florida, Gainesville, Florida
Clinical Professor of Medicine (Cardiology)
University of South Florida, Tampa, Florida

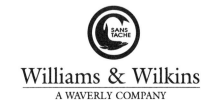

Williams & Wilkins
A WAVERLY COMPANY

BALTIMORE • PHILADELPHIA • LONDON • PARIS • BANGKOK
BUENOS AIRES • HONG KONG • MUNICH • SYDNEY • TOKYO • WROCLAW

Editor: Jonathan W. Pine, Jr.
Managing Editor: Lynn Johnston
Marketing Manager: Daniell T. Griffin
Production Coordinator: Raymond E. Reter
Copy Editor: Jeffrey S. Myers
Text and Cover Designer: Artech, Baltimore, Maryland
Illustration Planner: Lorraine Wrzosek
Typesetter: Peirce Graphic Services, Inc., Stuart, Florida
Printer & Binder: Mack Printing Group, Easton, Pennsylvania
Digitized Illustrations: Peirce Graphic Services, Inc., Stuart, Florida

Copyright © 1998 Williams & Wilkins

351 West Camden Street
Baltimore, Maryland 21201-2436 USA

Rose Tree Corporate Center
1400 North Providence Road
Building II, Suite 5025
Media, Pennsylvania 19063–2043 USA

All rights reserved. This book is protected by copyright. No part of this book may be reproduced in any form or by any means, including photocopying, or utilized by any information storage and retrieval system without written permission from the copyright owner.

Accurate indications, adverse reactions and dosage schedules for drugs are provided in this book, but it is possible that they may change. The reader is urged to review the package information data of the manufacturers of the medications mentioned.

Printed in the United States of America

First Edition 1990

Library of Congress Cataloging-in-Publication Data

Marriott, Henry J. L. (Henry Joseph Llewellyn), 1917–
    Pearls & pitfalls in electrocardiography : pithy, practical
pointers / Henry J. L. Marriott.–2nd ed.
        p.   cm.
    Includes bibliographical references and index.
    ISBN 0-683-30170-5
    1. Electrocardiography.   I. Title.
    [DNLM: 1. Electrocardiography.   WG 140 M359pa 1998]
RC683.5.E5M298 1998
616.1′2′07547–dc21
DNLM/DLC   97–13639
for Library of Congress   CIP

The publishers have made every effort to trace the copyright holders for borrowed material. If they have inadvertently overlooked any, they will be pleased to make the necessary arrangements at the first opportunity.

To purchase additional copies of this book, call our customer service department at **(800) 638-0672** or fax orders to **(800) 447-8438.** For other book services, including chapter reprints and large quantity sales, ask for the Special Sales department.

Canadian customers should call **(800) 665-1148,** or fax **(800) 665-0103.** For all other calls originating outside of the United States, please call **(410) 528-4223** or fax us at **(410) 528-8550.**

Visit Williams & Wilkins on the Internet: **http://www.wwilkins.com** or contact our customer service department at **custserv@wwilkins.com.** Williams & Wilkins customer service representatives are available from 8:30 am to 6:00 pm, EST, Monday through Friday, for telephone access.

98 99 00 01
2 3 4 5 6 7 8 9 10

PREFACE

With practice, interpretation of most ECGs is easy enough; but no matter how proficient you are, the accurate interpretation of some tracings remains difficult and sometimes impossible. We still have a lot to learn, and any "tricks of the trade" that simplify our task are well worth acquiring. In general, these stratagems take two forms: knowledge and use of clues that provide short cuts to the diagnosis ("pearls"), and awareness and avoidance of traps that can—and often do—deceive the unwary ("pitfalls").

An example of the sort of gimmick that helps to keep us out of trouble is the realization that there are many pairs of mutual mimics, and that whenever you see one of a known pair, you automatically think of its mimicking twin. For example, nonconducted atrial bigeminy can simulate sinus bradycardia to perfection; therefore, whenever you encounter sinus bradycardia you should automatically think of nonconducted atrial bigeminy and exclude it. Remember, the first step towards any diagnosis is to THINK OF IT!

"Pearls," to use an Oslerian phrase, are "burrs that stick in the memory." They condense in memorable form a diagnostic clue, often one that is not widely appreciated. A "pearl" is easily stored in the memory, a treasure carried without effort—like its material, oyster-borne counterpart!—and an appropriate tracing immediately triggers its recollection.

"Pitfalls" are unsuspected sources of error—footpads lying in wait to ambush the interpreter if he or she does not tread warily. Artifact that imitates atrial activity, concealed junctional extrasystoles mimicking type II AV block, and ventricular aberration masquerading as ectopy are examples of diagnostic pitfalls. To be aware is to beware!

But it is difficult to segregate pearls from pitfalls, because knowledge of a pitfall becomes a pearl when it enables the possessor of that knowledge to avoid the trap. And so, to avoid any attempt at artificial segregation, I decided to categorize the items according to the context to which they relate: arrhythmias, blocks, and 12-lead tracings. This encounters a minor snag because again there is unavoidable overlap. For example, a pacemaker is implanted for block but produces an arrhythmia; should it be classified in the section for block or arrhythmia? Or again, the concealed junctional extrasystole is an *arrhythmia,* but its chief importance is that it simulates *block*. Should it be classified in the section for block or arrhythmia?

I elected to classify the item under whatever came first: in the case of the pacemaker, block was obviously present before the pacemaker made its appearance, and therefore the items related to pacemakers are found in the section involving blocks.

This is not a textbook, and it is not a collection of rare birds. The sole criteria for inclusion are: (1) that the item is often either not known or misunderstood as determined from widespread encounters with cardiac personnel; and (2) that the item has practical value in helping to make the diagnosis, in helping one not to miss a diagnosis, or in preventing one from making the wrong diagnosis. Rarae aves are not excluded but each item is certainly practical. A knowledge of the contents will protect the beginner against some prevalent false doctrines and give one an effortless edge of sophistication beyond one's peers; and it will enable the cardiologist to hone his or her skill because the text contains many valuable pointers in topics where even experts have been known to founder.

St. Petersburg, Florida   Henry J. L. Marriott

NOTICES TO READER

Intervals, unless otherwise specified, are expressed in hundredths of a second, e.g., in Figure 6-C the parasystolic interval is 160 (i.e., 1.60 s).

The following **abbreviations** are of such common coinage that they will be used throughout the text without further explanation:

APB	=	atrial premature beat (or extrasystole)
A-V	=	atrioventricular
BBB	=	bundle-branch block
ECG	=	electrocardiogram
LBBB	=	left bundle-branch block
LV	=	left ventricle or ventricular
LVH	=	left ventricular hypertrophy
RBBB	=	right bundle-branch block
RV	=	right ventricle or ventricular
RVH	=	right ventricular hypertrophy
s	=	second
S-A	=	sino-atrial (or sinus)
VPB	=	ventricular premature beat (or extrasystole)
WPW	=	Wolff-Parkinson-White

CONTENTS

Part 1: Mostly Arrhythmias

Part 2: Unheavenly Twins

Part 3: Mostly Blocks

Part 4: 12-Lead Revelations

PART 1
MOSTLY ARRHYTHMIAS

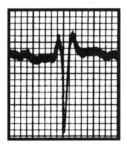

1 THE FIVE-POINT APPROACH

Most arrhythmias are easily diagnosed. It usually takes only a glance to recognize complete A-V block or atrial flutter with 4:1 A-V conduction. But if the arrhythmic mechanism is not immediately obvious, it is good to have a logical schema to turn to. More diagnoses are missed for lack of logic than because of ignorance.

Having observed countless interpreters—including myself—fail to make a correct diagnosis of some or other arrhythmic disturbance, and having analyzed what seemed to be the reasons for our failures, a system evolved that has proven invaluable in approaching the more obscure arrhythmia. If at first the arrhythmic mechanism is not obvious, proceed in five, logical, consecutive steps:

KNOW THE CAUSES

As in all medical diagnosis, the biggest step is to think of it. If we want to be experts, we must first know the causes of the problems we encounter. When faced with, for example, a difficult hemoptysis problem, the first step is to think of the causes of hemoptysis. Somewhere in our recitation of the causes, we will mention the diagnosis. It is no different with the arrhythmias—we must know the causes of the various disturbances of rhythm (1). Take, for example, bradycardia; there are only four causes of a regular bradycardia: sinus bradycardia, nonconducted atrial bigeminy, sinus block, and A-V block. Therefore, whenever we see a bradycardia the diagnosis must be one of those four.

Of course there are other bradycardias, e.g., idioventricular rhythm. But idioventricular rhythm is not a *cause* of bradycardia; it *always results from* one of the four just mentioned mechanisms.

MILK THE QRS

This is emphasized because the P wave has been unduly stressed in the past as the primary target. The informational treasure trove contained in the QRS is discussed in #11. Only after the ventricular complex has yielded up its secrets should the P wave be pursued.

CHERCHEZ LE P

At times the P wave undoubtedly holds the key and must be diligently sought and evaluated.

ESTABLISH RELATIONSHIPS

This is a very important step and refers to any relationships that can be recognized, not just the relationship of P to QRS. Its application is seen, for example, in Figure 19-B.

PINPOINT THE PRIMARY DIAGNOSIS

This is a must before initiating therapy. A-V dissociation, for example, is not a diagnosis, it is always secondary to one of four primary disturbances (see #38); and it is one of the four disturbances that merits treatment, if treatment is required.

If this systematic approach is adhered to whenever a difficult arrhythmic diagnosis is encountered, mistakes of omission and commission will be rare indeed.

REFERENCE

1. Marriott HJ. Practical Electrocardiography. 8th ed. Baltimore: Williams & Wilkins, 1988, p. 122.

2 Q WAVES IN ECTOPIC BEATS

At times, Q waves pathognomonic of myocardial infarction (MI), for reasons not fully understood, may show up better or only in *ectopic* ventricular beats. There may also be ST and T wave changes characteristic of MI.

Figure 2-A shows an example in an ophthalmologist who had an MI 2 years before this tracing was taken. The conducted sinus beats show no sign of pathologic Q waves, whereas the VPBs all manifest a wide Q wave characteristic of myocardial necrosis. For the Q wave to be significant, it must be followed by a sizeable R wave—a QS complex is not enough(1–3).

Figure 2-B is from another patient with an acute anteroseptal infarction. The QRS of his sinus beats show no evidence of MI, whereas the ventricular extrasystole not only possesses a deep wide Q wave, but the ST segment is also elevated and the T wave inverted. Figure 2-C presents yet another example.

But perhaps the context in which the extrasystolic configuration can be most useful is when, in the presence of LBBB, the diagnosis of acute MI is uncertain and a stray VPB proclaims the infarction with typical QRS-T changes (Fig. 2-D).

Such Q waves, however, are not the monopoly of infarction; occasionally a patient with hypertrophic cardiomyopathy can manifests similar Q waves only in his ectopic beats (4).

REFERENCES

1. Bisteni A, et al. Ventricular premature beats in the diagnosis of myocardial infarction. Br Heart J 1961;23:521.
2. Benchimol A, et al. The ventricular premature contraction. Its place in the diagnosis of ischemic heart disease. Am Heart J 1963;65:334.
3. Wahl JM, et al. Limitations of premature ventricular complex morphology in the diagnosis of myocardial infarction. J Electrocardiol 1986;19:131.
4. Abdulla AM, et al. Value of ventricular complex (VPC) morphology in the diagnosis of hypertrophic cardiomyopathy. J Electrocardiol 1983;16:73.

FIG. 2.

A – From a 49-year-old ophthalmologist who had an anterior infarction 2 years previously. The sinus bradycardia is punctuated by interpolated VPBs; those in the top strip and the second in the bottom strip have infarction-like Q waves followed by significant R waves. The QS configuration, as seen in the first VPB in the bottom strip, is not considered suggestive of infarction. (Reproduced from Marriott HJ. Practical Electrocardiography. 8th ed. Baltimore: Williams & Wilkins, 1988.)

B – The QRSs of the sinus beats in another patient show nothing suspicious of infarction although their ST segments are distinctly elevated; but all of the several premature beats manifest the wide Q waves, ST segment elevation and inverted T waves typical of acute infarction.

C – With QS complexes from V1-V4, an anterior infarction is highly suspect (see also #59). The shape of the ventricular ectopic beat in V1 (wide Q, followed by sizeable R wave and inverted T wave) and to a less extent the configuration in V2 and V3, provides strong confirmation of the infarction.

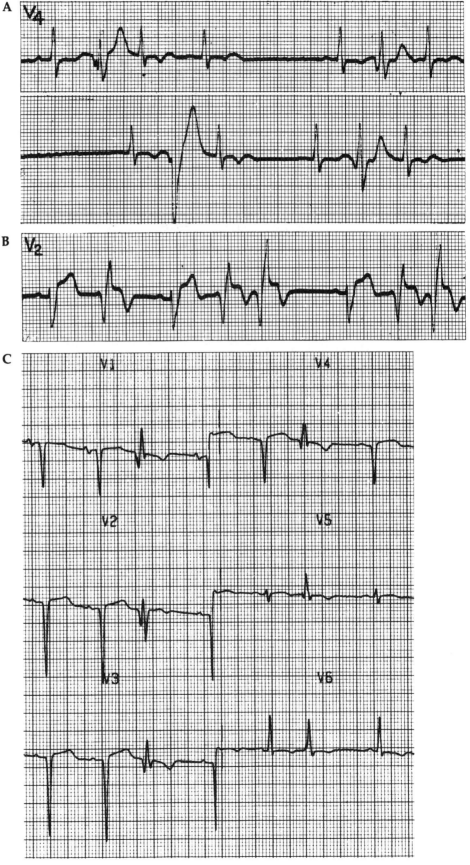

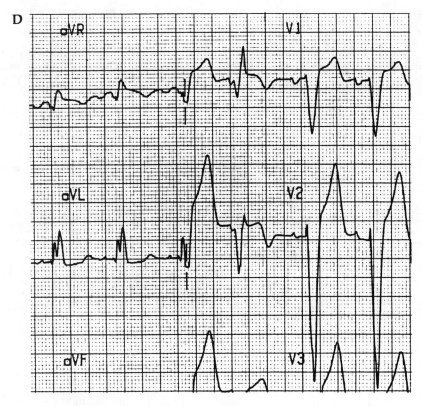

FIG. 2. *(continued)*

D – This excerpt from a 12-lead tracing of LBBB presents six consecutive beats, the fourth of which is a VPB. From the beats manifesting BBB, a diagnosis of acute infarction cannot be made (though the Q wave in AVL bespeaks an infarction at some time—see #49); but the changes in the VPB—deep, wide Q wave, ST elevation and inverted T wave—are clearly diagnostic.

3 SIMULATED VENTRICULAR BIGEMINY

Whenever you see what you think is ventricular bigeminy in the presence of atrial flutter, be sure to exclude alternating 2:1 and 4:1 conduction with ventricular aberration of the beats that end the shorter cycles.

This can be an important booby trap in patients receiving digitalis for control of the ventricular rate during atrial flutter. A patient with atrial flutter and 2:1 conduction, for example, has a ventricular rate of 150/min. The patient is started on a digitalis preparation, probably digoxin, with the idea of slowing the ventricular response and perhaps converting the atrial flutter. On the way to achieving a goal of 4:1 conduction and therefore a normal ventricular rate of 75/min, regardless of the drug used (e.g., digitalis, propranolol, or verapamil), the patient is likely to develop a Wenckebach in the A-V junction below the 2:1 "filter";

and if the Wenckebach has a ratio of 3:2, the result will be alternating 2:1 and 4:1 A-V conduction (Fig. 3-A). As seen in Figure 3-A, note the long F-R intervals. Besoain-Santander, Pick and Langendorf long ago observed that, in atrial flutter, the conduction time (F-R interval) was usually between 0.26 and 0.46 s because of the rapid, repetitive partial penetration of the junction (concealed conduction, see also #39)(1).

Now if aberration develops in the beats that end the shorter cycles (Fig. 3-B), ventricular bigeminy is simulated. And if digoxin is what the patient is receiving, then digitalis intoxication is naturally suspected and may be diagnosed; whereupon the digoxin is discontinued, yet the patient needs more of the drug to further reduce the conduction ratio to 4:1.

REFERENCE

1. Besoain-Santander M, Pick A, Langendorf R. A-V conduction in auricular flutter. Circulation, 1950;2:604

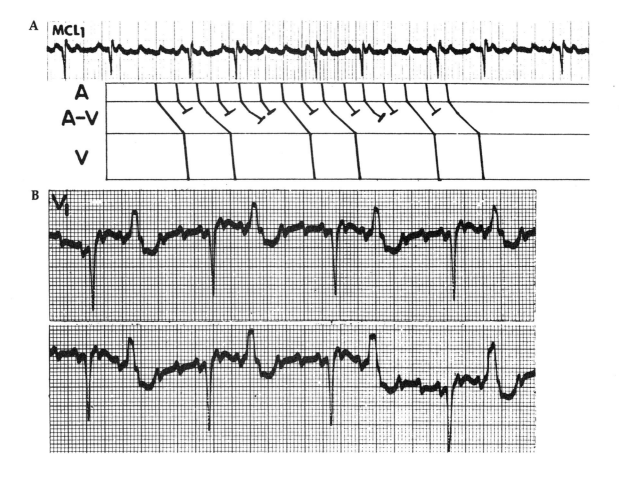

FIG. 3.

A – The laddergram portrays the usual mechanism when, during atrial flutter, the ventricular complexes are arranged in pairs. Against a background of 2:1 conduction, 3:2 Wenckebach conduction develops at a level below the 2:1 "filter" that results in alternating 2:1 and 4:1 A-V conduction.

B – Atrial flutter with probable alternating 2:1 and 4:1 conduction with RBBB aberration of the beats ending the shorter cycles.

4 THE BIX RULE

This clue is named after Harold Bix, the Viennese cardiologist who practiced in Baltimore and had an encyclopedic knowledge of arrhythmias, and who drew attention to the fact that if you are dealing with a supraventricular tachycardia in which the visible P′ wave is situated midway between the ventricular complexes, the probability is that there are P waves lurking within the QRS complexes. In other words, there is usually an atrial tachyarrhythmia (tachycardia or flutter) with 2:1 A-V conduction. This is well shown in Figure 4-A in which the top strip shows a supraventricular tachycardia with P′ waves halfway between the ventricular complexes. In the bottom strip, a spontaneous change in A-V conduction exposes the lurking P′ waves and confirms that the atrial rate is twice as fast as it appeared in the top strip. Figures 4-B and 4-C present additional examples of this phenomenon.

Recognition of this situation is of great therapeutic importance. It is better to be forewarned that the ratio is 2:1 because, if the atrial rate were to slow—for instance under the influence of ill-advised quinidine (Fig. 4-C) or procainamide—there would be a real risk of 1:1 conduction developing with a dangerously rapid ventricular response. It is better to be alert to this possibility ahead of time and not be taken by surprise.

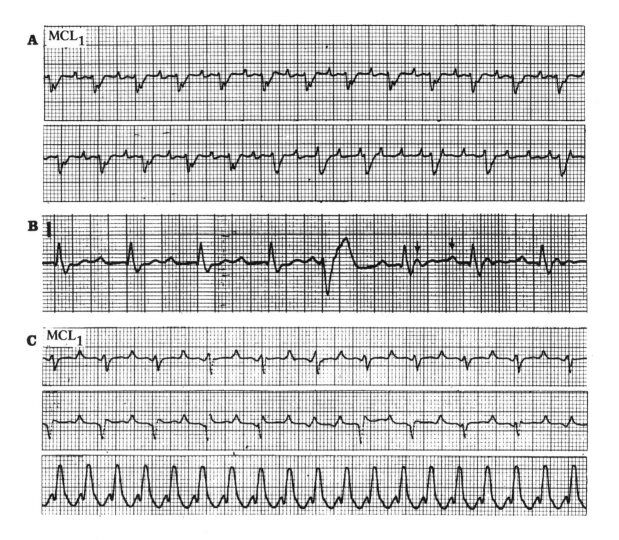

FIG. 4.

A – Strips are continuous. In the top strip, atrial tachycardia is present with consistent 2:1 conduction, the visible P′ wave being halfway between the QRS complexes. In the bottom strip, the A-V conduction ratio spontaneously changes revealing the hitherto hidden P′ waves.

B – After several beats that appear to represent sinus rhythm with first degree A-V block, in which the P wave is approximately midway between the QRS complexes, a VPB intrudes. As a result, the next atrial impulse is conducted after a longer R-P interval with a consequently shorter P-R interval (see #29 and 30). This shorter P-R interval causes the next P wave to emerge from under cover of the QRS and reveals the twice–as–fast atrial rate (arrows).

C – **Top strip:** Atrial tachycardia with consistent 2:1 A-V conduction. **Middle strip:** After several doses of digoxin, occasional 4:1 A-V conduction ratios occurred and the patient was inappropriately started on quinidine. **Bottom strip:** Due to the quinidine, the atrial rate decreased from 210/min to 195/min and 1:1 A-V conduction and RBBB developed; the patient was then treated for hours for ventricular tachycardia (Reproduced from Marriott HJ. Practical Electrocardiography. 8th ed. Baltimore: Williams & Wilkins, 1988. p. 255.).

5 DECEPTIVE P-WAVE POLARITY

The polarity of P waves is not always immediately obvious. If you look at the junctional tachycardia depicted in Figure 5-A, and concentrate on the atrial activity that follows every alternate QRS complex in the top strip; and if you are familiar with the phenomenon of retrograde conduction, you will almost certainly think at first that the P waves are inverted and therefore retrograde.

Actually, they are upright sinus P waves. You can see one of these sinus P waves and its unequivocally positive polarity if you look just in front of the last QRS in the bottom strip. Now if you look back at the top strip and compare consecutive ST segments, it becomes obvious that the alternating deformity is due to a positive bump and not to a negative trough. The negative effect is of course caused by the downstroke of the positive P wave.

Take note that mistaking the polarity of these P waves is an error that the unsophisticated, unprejudiced eye could not make; it is only because one has knowledge of retrograde conduction that the mistake can be made. "When a man has special knowledge . . . it rather encourages him to seek a complex explanation when a simple one is at hand (1)."

The message here is that one must learn to superimpose corresponding segments of the tracing (Fig. 5-B) in the mind's eye in order to discern the polarity of deforming P waves.

REFERENCE

1. Sherlock Holmes in Abbey Grange.

5

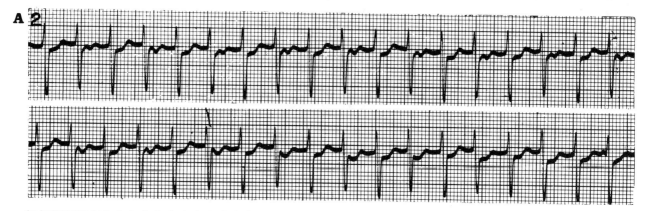

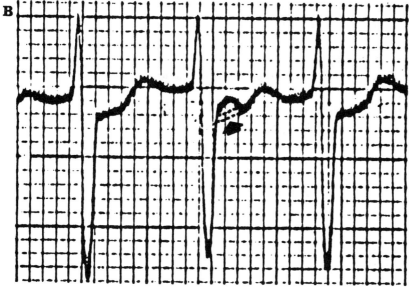

FIG. 5.

A – Junctional tachycardia dissociated from sinus rhythm at almost exactly half the rate. The downstroke of the sinus P wave, landing after every alternate QRS, produces the impression of a negative deflection and thus erroneously suggests retrograde conduction. In the bottom strip, the sinus P wave gradually disappears within the QRS, finally emerging just in front of the last QRS.

B – To restore the deformed ST segment, it is necessary to shave off a positive bump (arrow)—not eliminate the seemingly negative trough.

6 PARASYSTOLE'S LOST MYSTIQUE

Parasystole is an arrhythmia often regarded as complex and mysterious; yet parasystole is nothing but a natural fixed-rate pacemaker, and no one has difficulty understanding the behavior of a fixed-rate (VOO) pacemaker: it continues to fire relentlessly regardless of circumnavigating sinus or other impulses. When the pacing stimulus prods the myocardium at a time that the muscle is not refractory, the pacemaker "captures" the ventricles and produces a paced QRS complex. When it discharges its stimulus at a time when the myocardium is refractory, the stimulus artifact is recorded but does not evoke a ventricular complex. If the artificial stimulus activates the myocardium at a moment when the descending sinus (or other) impulse is also invading the ventricular myocardium, a fusion beat results. Regardless of what other impulses are activating the ventricles, the pacing stimulus is delivered and the stimulus artifact is recorded with monotonous and uninterrupted regularity. Thus, the intervals between paced beats always equal the automatic cycle of the pacemaker or are multiples thereof.

Parasystole shares with the fixed-rate pacemaker its two outstanding characteristics: nondisturbable and independent. The only difference between them is that the parasystolic rhythm does not inscribe stimulus artifacts in the record.

Parasystole (Figs. 6-A to C) is therefore recognized by the fact that its ectopic beats follow the preceding sinus beats at *varying* intervals (so-called "coupling" intervals)—evidence of independence; and that the cycles between consecutive ectopic beats are either the basic parasystolic cycle or multiples thereof—evidence of its nondisturbable characteristic. This is usually expressed by stating that the interectopic intervals all have a common denominator, i.e., the parasystolic cycle.

Although the parasystolic discharge is usually absolutely regular, we now know that the parasystolic pacemaker can be modulated by the electrotonic effects of sinus impulses that knock at the closed (protective) door, but cannot enter. They cannot discharge the center but they can influence it to beat somewhat ahead or behind its regular schedule (1,2).

REFERENCES

1. Castellanos A, et al. Annihilation, entrainment and modulation of ventricular parasystolic rhythms. Am J Cardiol 1984;54;317.
2. Castellanos A, et al. Concealment of manifest, and exposure of concealed ventricular parasystole produced by isoproterenol. Am J Cardiol 1985;55:1344.

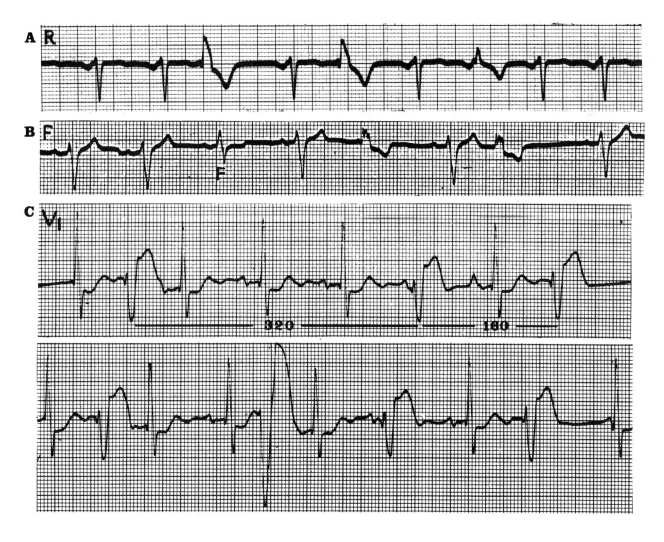

FIG. 6.

A – Although this rhythm strip is much too short to make the definitive diagnosis of parasystole, it shows the cardinal characteristics of that arrhythmia with great clarity. While the interval between the ectopic beats and the preceding sinus beats ("coupling" interval) progressively lengthens, the interectopic intervals are precisely equal; and the third ectopic impulse, arrives as it does after the next sinus P wave, producing fusion.

B – This strip is also too short for certain diagnosis, but again it shows the cardinal features of parasystole. The first parasystolic beat, landing after the P wave, produces fusion (F), while the subsequent beats have progressively shortening "coupling" intervals.

C – Ventricular parasystole. Second, sixth, and eighth beats in the top strip, and second, seventh, and ninth in the bottom strip are parasystolic. The fifth beat in the bottom strip is an interpolated extrasystole. The cycle of the parasystolic rhythm (160) is indicated by the interval between the second and third parasystolic beats in each strip. The interval between first and second parasystolic beats in both strips is exactly twice this cycle. Thus, while the "coupling" intervals markedly vary, the parasystolic cycle remains constant. After the final parasystolic beat, the returning cycle ends with junctional escape.

7 DEVIANT FUSION BEATS

Fusion beats, when accurately identified, may be valuable diagnostic props. Because the vast majority of fusion beats result from the collision of supraventricular and ventricular impulses within the ventricular myocardium, the fusion beats resulting from this usual combination have a QRS morphology and duration that is intermediate between the shape and width of the "component" complexes. If, for example, a patient's QRS during sinus rhythm has a duration of 0.07 s, and the QRS of the ectopic rhythm has a duration of 0.14 s, then all of the fusion complexes will (A) have a duration somewhere between 0.07 and 0.14 s and (B) bear some recognizable resemblance to one or both of these "component" complexes. The resulting duration and shape depend upon the contribution of each impulse to the fusing form.

There are two exceptions to these general rules, situations that have been neatly epigrammed by Schamroth: "Two wrongs sometimes make a right!"

Exception 1: If a patient with BBB has an ectopic focus on the same side as the BBB, and the ectopic focus fires at the same moment that the descending sinus impulse enters the contralateral ventricle, the two ventricles will be activated simultaneously and the resulting fusion complex will be normally narrow and unlike either of the component QRSs (Figs. 7-A to D).

Exception 2: If, in the presence of complete A-V block, there happens to be an alert idioventricular pacemaker in each ventricle, and if the two of them fire simultaneously, the fusion resulting from their simultaneous discharge will also produce a complex narrower than, and not at all resembling, either of the individual idioventricular complexes (Fig. 7-E).

FIG. 7.

A – The four strips are continuous. Fusion between an idioventricular pacemaker in the *right* ventricle and junctional rhythm with *right* BBB. Beats two through five in the top strip, and the first beat in the second strip, represent the idioventricular rhythm from the right ventricle. With the second beat in the second strip, fusion begins and its most obvious sign is lowering of the T wave. With successive beats the T wave becomes lower and the QRS narrower until the first beat in the third strip has the appearance of a normally conducted QRS. As the junctional rhythm makes a greater and greater contribution to the fusion beats, the pattern of RBBB progressively evolves and persists through the bottom strip.

B – Schamroth's neat diagram of three forms of conduction seen when a *right* ventricular pacemaker competes with sinus rhythm in the presence of *right* BBB. Beats one and three: sinus conducted with RBBB. Beat four: right ventricular ectopic. Beat two: fusion between right ventricular ectopic and conducted sinus impulse in presence of RBBB producing normally narrow QRS complex.

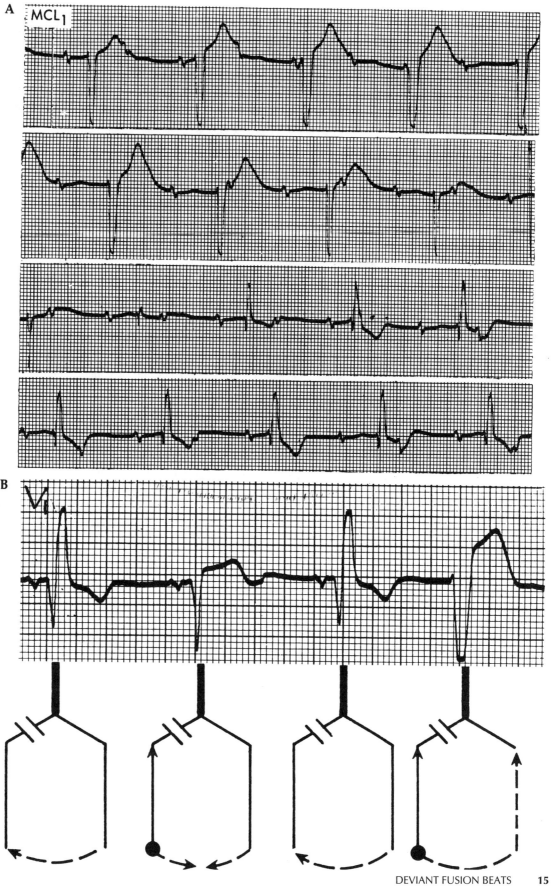

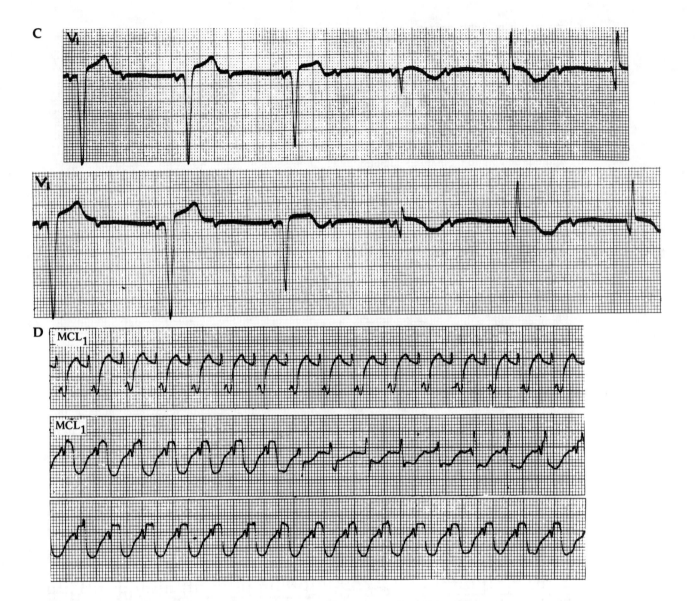

FIG. 7. *(continued)*

C – The two strips are not continuous. Fusion between an idioventricular rhythm in the *left* ventricle and sinus rhythm with *left* BBB. Both strips begin with 2:1 type II A-V block and LBBB. The fifth and sixth beats in each strip are idioventricular beats from the left ventricle. Third and fourth beats in each strip are fusion beats showing intermediate shapes. Note particularly the fourth beat in the top strip, which has the appearance of a completely normal QRS.

D – *Left* ventricular tachycardia in the presence of *left* BBB, producing narrow fusion beats. **Top strip:** Sinus tachycardia with LBBB. **Bottom two strips** (which are continuous): Left ventricular tachycardia appears and, after the seventh beat, a series of narrow fusion beats develop with gradual widening toward the end of the strip—the P wave approaches the QRS, the P-R interval shortens, and the ectopic impulse contributes more and more to the fusion complexes. The first beat in the bottom strip is the last of the fusion beats, whereupon the "pure" left ventricular tachycardia resumes.

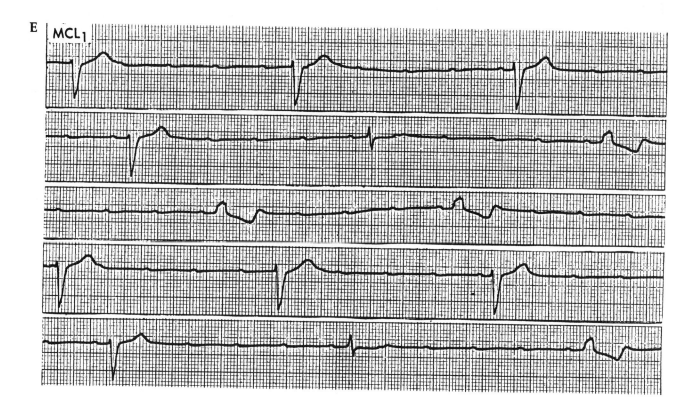

FIG. 7. *(continued)*

E – The strips are continuous. Sinus tachycardia with complete A-V block and escape rhythms from both ventricles at a rate of 21–22/min. The three beats in the **top strip** are from the RV (or they *may* be junctional with
LBBB), while the two beats in the **third strip** are from the LV. The first beat in the **second strip** is RV, the
third is LV, and the one midway between them is a fusion beat; the fifth strip is a replay of the second. The fusion beats are narrow because they result from the simultaneous activation of both ventricles by their respective pacemakers (Reproduced from Marriott HJ. Practical Electrocardiography. 8th ed. Baltimore: Williams &
Wilkins, 1988. p. 318.).

8 VENTRICULAR TACHYCARDIA AND P WAVES

Many authorities claim that the way to diagnose ventricular tachycardia (VT) is to detect independent atrial activity. It is undoubtedly true that IF you find independent P waves (or any other evidence of A-V dissociation, such as variation in intensity of the first heart sound, irregular cannon waves in the neck, etc.) in the presence of a wide-QRS tachycardia, it is extremely strong evidence in favor of VT (Fig. 8-A). But as the main diagnostic prop, A-V dissociation is a broken reed.

This is so because in about half of the VTs there are no *independent* P waves; about 45% have retrograde conduction to the atria, and 5% are associated with atrial fibrillation. In a recent series of 100 proven VTs, only 27 had independent P waves (1). Therefore, depending on uncovering independent P waves to make the diagnosis is like refusing to call the writhing reptile a snake until you hear the rattle! Moreover, of the approximately 50% who have independent atrial activity, you will be able to find P waves in the clinical tracing in only about half—to uncover the atrial activity in the others will require an additional maneuver, such as passing an esophageal electrode or an atrial wire, which is uncomfortable and may be dangerous for the patient.

It is usually in the less rapid tachycardias, where diagnosis is less urgent, that independent P waves are likely to be found (e.g., Fig. 8-A); and there is, of course, the rare exception of the patient with junctional tachycardia and BBB with no retrograde conduction and therefore dissociated atria (Fig. 8-B).

REFERENCE

1. Niazi I, et al. Reevaluation of surface ECG criteria for the diagnosis of wide QRS tachycardia. Circulation 1987;76(Suppl 4):412.

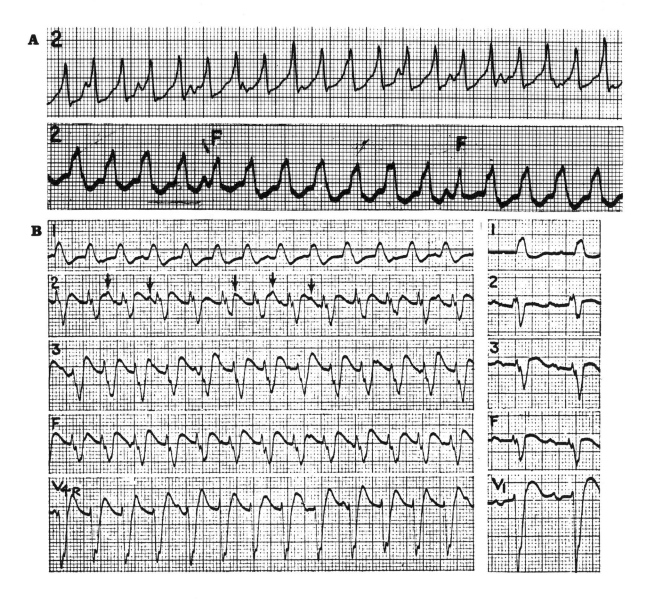

FIG. 8.

A – Two examples of ventricular tachycardia with clearly visible independent P waves. **Top strip:** Ventricular rate 190/min, and no evident fusion beats. **Bottom strip:** Ventricular rate 155/min, with two obvious fusion beats (F). This is about the fastest rate at which fusion beats are likely to be seen.

B – An example of junctional tachycardia with LBBB and no retrograde conduction, and therefore independent P waves (arrows). **Right panel:** Unchanged QRS morphology during conducted sinus rhythm—confirmation that the tachycardia was supraventricular.

9 FRAILTY OF LEAD 2

In the days before the diagnostic value of QRS morphology was appreciated, lead 2 was the standard lead for studying arrhythmias—probably because it was a lead in which P waves were usually prominent. With increasing knowledge and appreciation of QRS morphology (see #11), a right chest lead, such as V1 or MCL1, has become deservedly popular and preferred.

A good reason for not using lead 2 to monitor is that all four of the common causes of wide QRSs—RBBB, LBBB, RV ectopy and LV ectopy—can look virtually identical in this lead (Fig. 9-A).

Another reason is that atrial activity may be seen best, or only, in a right chest lead (Figs. 9-B and C). In the only study in which the diagnostic capability of lead 2 was compared with that of chest leads, the correct diagnosis was made from V1, MCL1, V6 or MCL6 in 74%–81% of 121 wide-QRS tachycardias, whereas the diagnostic yield from lead 2 was only 34%(1).

REFERENCE

1. Drew BJ, Scheinman MM. Value of electrocardiographic leads MCL1, MCL6 and other selected leads in the diagnosis of wide QRS complex tachycardia. JACC 1991;18:1025.

FIG. 9.

A – The four main causes of widened QRS complexes: (1) RBBB, (2) LBBB, (3) RV tachycardia, and (4) LV tachycardia. Despite the great morphologic variety in V1, in all four conditions lead 2 can present a QS complex.

B – Atrial tachycardia with 2:1 A-V conduction. Note that the P′ waves are readily identified in V1 but not in lead 2.

C – This is from the same patient as Figure 3-B; the flutter waves that were so obvious in lead V1 are quite invisible in lead 2. The rhythm here looks like junctional with ventricular bigeminy; but combining the information obtained from both leads (V1 and 2), the diagnosis is apparently atrial flutter with alternating 4:1 and 2:1 conduction, with RBBB and left anterior hemiblock aberration of the beats ending the shorter cycles.

D – A further example of the invisibility of atrial activity in lead 2 with easy recognition in V1. And another example of the mechanism often seen in atrial flutter; 2:1 "filtering" of the flutter impulses at an upper level in the AV junction with a Wenckebach of varied ratio developing in the beats that get through the "filter" on their way to the ventricles (see other examples in #3A and #31B).

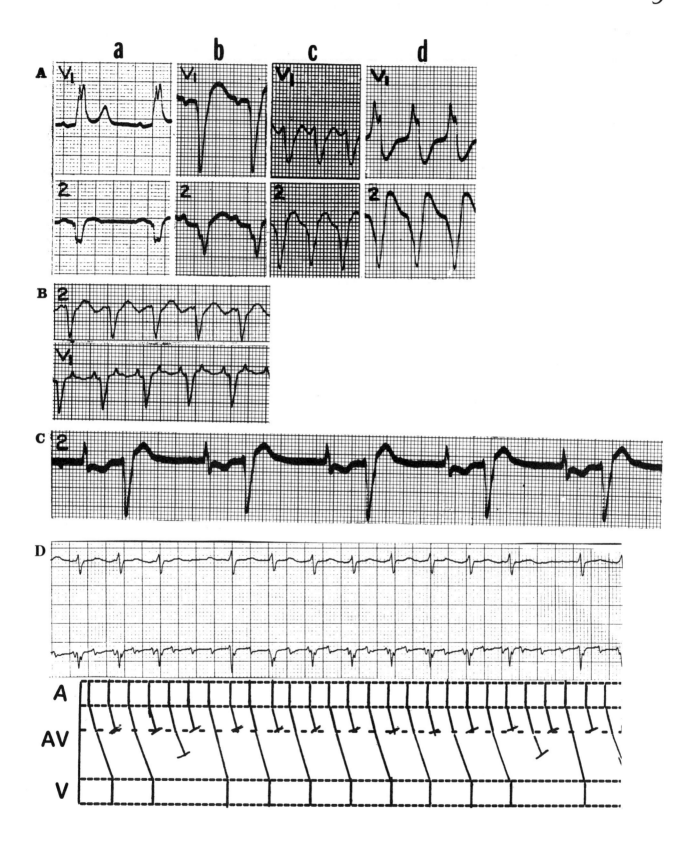

9

10 ASHMAN'S PHENOMENON

The so-called Ashman phenomenon often causes diagnostic confusion. In 1947, Gouaux and Ashman drew attention to the fact that, during atrial fibrillation, when a relatively long cycle was followed by a relatively short one, the beat that ended the shorter cycle often developed BBB aberration[1] (Figs. 10-A to C). The reason for this is clear. The refractory period of the ventricular conduction system varies with the rate and is therefore proportional to the preceding cycle; a longer cycle lengthens the ensuing refractory period, and if a considerably shorter cycle follows, the beat ending it is likely to be caught in the lengthened refractory period of one of the bundle branches.

Those who have heard of the phenomenon appear to assume that a long-short cycle sequence ending with an anomalous beat is therefore aberrant. Unfortunately, according to the "rule of bigeminy," a lengthened cycle tends to precipitate a ventricular extrasystole (Figs. 10-D and E); therefore, a long-short cycle sequence ending with an anomalous beat cannot be used to favor either aberration or ectopy because it favors both[2]! Consequently, when differentiating between aberration or ectopy, one depends heavily on the QRS morphology (see #11).

A caveat: comparison of cycle-sequences is not infallible because of the unpredictability of concealed conduction into a bundle branch. If one of the recent fibrillatory impulses happens to gain access to the right bundle branch, for example, but fails to reach the ventricular myocardium, a succeeding impulse (that manages to reach the ventricles) may find the invaded bundle branch refractory and, regardless of the preceding cycle length, be conducted with RBBB aberration.

REFERENCES

1. Gouaux JL, Ashman R. Auricular fibrillation with aberration simulating ventricular paroxysmal tachycardia. Am Heart J 1947;34:366.
2. Langendorf R, et al. Mechanisms of intermittent ventricular bigeminy. I. Appearance of ectopic beats dependent upon the length of the ventricular cycle, the "rule of bigeminy." Circulation 1955;11:442.

FIG. 10.

A to C – Three examples of the "Ashman phenomenon" characterized by RBBB aberration. Note in each example that the aberrant beat ends a short cycle preceded by the longest ventricular cycle in the strip. Compare with D and E where the longest cycle precipitates a ventricular extrasystole.

D – The "rule of bigeminy" at work. Atrial fibrillation is present and a marked lengthening of the ventricular cycle precipitates a ventricular extrasystole.

E – After three sinus beats, an APB by suppressing the sinus node ("overdrive" suppression) lengthens the next ventricular cycle enough to precipitate a run of ventricular bigeminy.

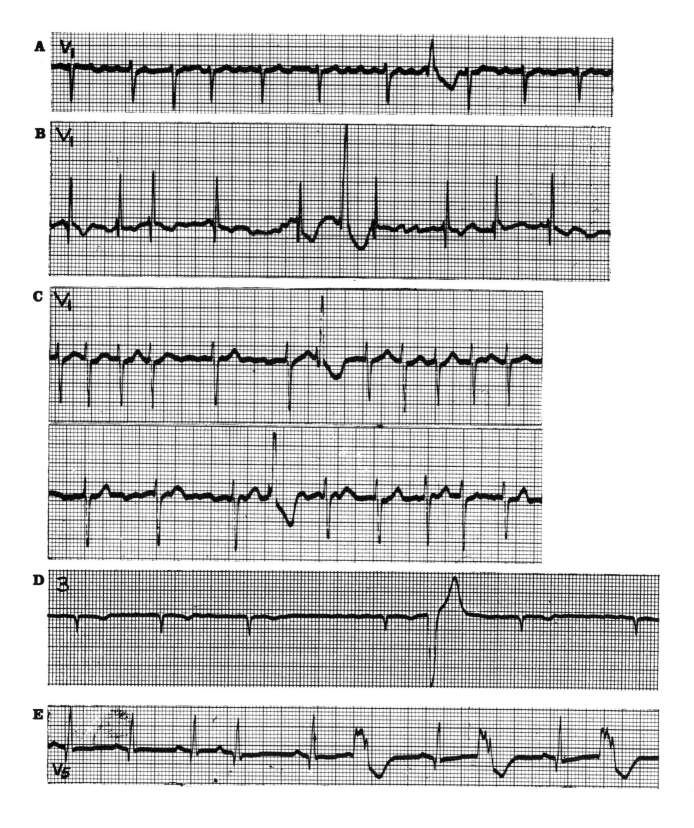

10

11 THE SHAPE OF THINGS

Judging by the inability of both physicians and critical care nurses to recognize the shape of ventricular ectopy, the information contained in this item should prove not only diagnostically rewarding, but also lifesaving (1–5).

The diagnostic pendulum in critical care has experienced an unexplained swing over the past decade or two. Fifteen years ago it was commonplace for a run of aberrant ventricular conduction to be misdiagnosed as ventricular tachycardia (VT) for which lidocaine was routinely administered. If the underlying rhythm was atrial fibrillation or atrial flutter, this usually led to a lengthening and acceleration of the runs of aberration, but usually no great harm was done. But the fashion has changed: today, the vogue seems to be an irresistible urge to call VT supraventricular with aberration—with the unfortunate result that verapamil is frequently given, sometimes with disastrous results (2–4). Most of the time this dangerous mistake is easily avoidable if the following precepts are observed:

PLAY THE ODDS

In 200 consecutive wide-QRS tachycardias, Wellens found 164 were ventricular, 30 were supraventricular with BBB, five were supraventricular with anterograde conduction over an accessory pathway, and one was supraventricular with conduction via a Mahaim fiber (6). Therefore, when faced with a wide-QRS tachycardia, it seems that the odds in favor of ventricular are approximately 5:1.

ASK THE RIGHT QUESTIONS

Akhtar and colleagues claim that if the answer to the following two questions is "yes," the diagnosis is almost invariably VT(7). (1) Have you ever had a heart attack? (2) Did the fast heart beating begin only after the heart attack?

DON'T BELIEVE THAT VT CANNOT BE WELL TOLERATED

The fact is that VT is often well tolerated for hours (1–2). The three factors that are more important than the origin of the tachycardia in determining hemodynamic tolerance are (1) the rate, (2) the size of the heart and (3) the presence and severity of any additional insult (e.g., myocardial infarction, digitalis intoxication, uremia, etc.).

DON'T DEPEND ON LEAD 2

Unfortunately, lead 2, which has been a popular monitoring lead, is one of the worst. One reason for this is that, as we saw in #9, it can look alike in all four of the common situations producing a wide QRS: LBBB, RBBB, RV ectopy and LV ectopy (Fig. 9-A).

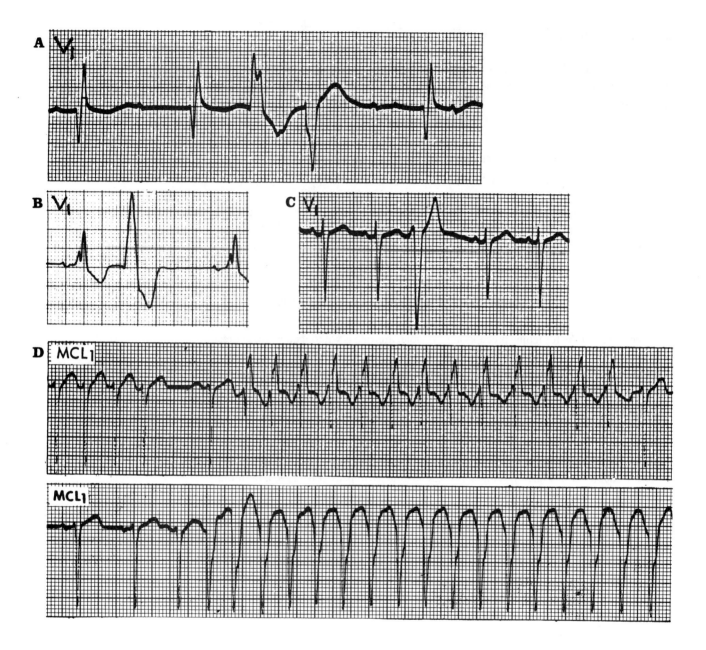

FIG. 11.

A – Here, side by side, *the* most typical shape of first LV and then RV ectopy is seen. The LV extrasystole is positive, with a taller left peak ("rabbit-ear"), whereas the RV extrasystole is negative with slurring of the downstroke to produce a late nadir (>0.07 s).

B – The LV extrasystole presents a single, symmetrical peak. The sinus beats are conducted with RBBB.

C – The RV extrasystole reaches a delayed nadir (>0.07 s), because of an initial wide r wave.

D – The **upper panel** shows the beginning of a supraventricular tachycardia with RBBB aberration; note the typical rSR′ pattern of RBBB. The **lower panel** shows the beginning of a run of supraventricular tachycardia with LBBB aberration; note the slick downstroke reaching an early nadir, with slurring on the upstroke. Contrast this with the pattern of RV ectopy in Figures 11-A and 11-C.

11

DON'T DEPEND ON IRREGULARITY

For years it has been taught that VT is usually irregular, whereas supraventricular tachycardia is regular. The fact is that although more than 90% of supraventricular tachycardias are absolutely regular, about 78% of VTs are also regular (8). Therefore, in any given case the presence or absence of regularity is of little assistance.

DON'T DEPEND UPON INDEPENDENT ATRIAL ACTIVITY TO MAKE THE DIAGNOSIS OF VT

Many people emphasize, and overemphasize, the importance of independent atrial activity to recognize VT. This has already been fully discussed in #8. The fact is, if you can't diagnose VT unless there is evidence of independent atria, you will miss at least half of them.

KNOW THE SUGGESTIVE QRS MORPHOLOGY AND POLARITY

Although all of the foregoing precepts are valuable, this one is without question of greatest value. If you are thoroughly familiar with the usual patterns of ectopy and aberration, you should be able to make an accurate diagnosis with considerable confidence in at least 85% of wide-QRS tachycardias (9). There is no other method that can achieve such accuracy except intracardiac electrophysiologic studies. The following clues are invaluable and should be memorized by everyone likely to encounter an urgent tachycardia (6–18).

In V1 (or MCL1): The following configurations favor ventricular ectopy: taller left peak ("rabbit ear") (Figs. 11-A and E), single symmetrical peak (Fig. 11-B), fat initial r wave (Fig. 11-C) or slurred downstroke (Fig. 11-A) to late nadir. The following configurations favor aberrant ventricular conduction: triphasic (rSR′ or some variant thereof) RBBB pattern (Fig. 11-D upper panel), LBBB pattern with sheer downstroke to early nadir (Fig. 11-D lower panel).
In V6 (or MCL6). The following configurations favor ventricular ectopy: rS (Fig. 11-F) or QS (Fig. 11-E); S wave or QS deeper than 15 mm (Figs. 11-E and F). A triphasic (qRs) RBBB pattern (Figs. 11-F and G) strongly favors aberration.
Limb leads. An axis in "no-man's land" (−90 to −180 degrees) (Fig. 11-E) strongly favors ventricular ectopy.
V leads. Concordance (i.e., all complexes either positive or negative from V1 to V6) favors ventricular ectopy(Fig. 11-H). Ventricular ectopy is also favored if there are no diphasic RS complexes in any of the V leads; or if, in the presence of RS complexes, it requires more than 0.10 s to reach the S nadir in any one of them (19,20).
Global QRS. If the 12-lead QRS pattern does not resemble either form of bundle branch block (Fig. 11-E), ventricular ectopy is strongly favored.

If all of the above precepts and clues are known and heeded, the misdiagnosis of a wide-QRS tachycardia should be rare.

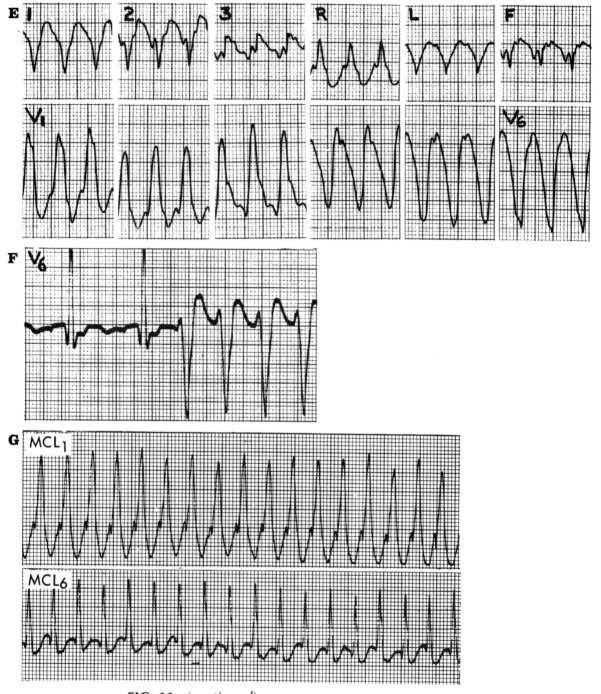

FIG. 11. *(continued)*

E – A 12-lead recording of a VT. Characteristic features include an axis in "no-man's land," early peak with slurring on the downstroke in V1, and QS complex deeper than 15 mm in V6.

F – After two supraventricular beats manifesting the qRs contour of RBBB, a paroxysm of VT begins with classical rS pattern and S wave 23 mm deep. (Reproduced from Marriott HJ. Practical Electrocardiography. 8th ed. Baltimore: Williams & Wilkins, 1988.)

G – Illustration of the diagnostic usefulness of the qRs pattern in MCL6 when the pattern is ambivalent in MCL1. (Reproduced from Marriott HJ. Practical Electrocardiography. 8th ed. Baltimore: Williams & Wilkins, 1988.)

11

REFERENCES

1. Morady F, et al. A prevalent misconception regarding wide-complex tachycardia. JAMA 1985;254:2790.
2. Dancy M, Camm AJ, Ward D. Misdiagnosis of chronic recurrent ventricular tachycardia. Lancet 1985;2:320.
3. Stewart RB, Bardy GH, Greene HL. Wide complex tachycardia: misdiagnosis and outcome after emergent therapy. Ann Intern Med 1986;104:766.
4. Switzer DF, et al. Dire consequences of verapamil administration for wide QRS tachycardias. Circulation 1986;74(Suppl 2):105.
5. Cooper J, Marriott HJ. Why are so many critical care nurses unable to recognize ventricular tachycardia in the 12-lead electrocardiogram? Heart Lung 1989;18:243.
6. Wellens HJ, Brugada P. Diagnosis of ventricular tachycardia from the 12-lead electrocardiogram. Cardiol Clin 1987;5:511.
7. Tchou P, et al. Useful clinical criteria for the diagnosis of ventricular tachycardia. Am J Med 1988;84:53–56.
8. Wellens HJ, Bar FW, Lie KI. The value of the electrocardiogram in the differential diagnosis of a tachycardia with a widened QRS complex. Am J Med 1978;64:27.
9. Wellens HJ, et al. The differentiation between ventricular tachycardia and supraventricular tachycardia with aberrant conduction: the value of the 12-lead electrocardiogram, in What's new in electrocardiography, Wellens HJ, Kulbertus HE, eds. Boston: Martinus Nijhoff. 1981 pp 184–199.
10. Sandler IA, Marriott HJ. The differential morphology of anomalous ventricular complexes of RBBB-type in lead V1: ventricular ectopy versus aberration. Circulation 1965;31:551.
11. Marriott HJ. Differential diagnosis of supraventricular and ventricular tachycardia. Geriatrics 1970;25:91.
12. Vera Z, et al. His bundle electrography for evaluation of criteria in differentiating ventricular ectopy from aberrance in atrial fibrillation Circulation. 1972;45(Suppl 2):90.
13. Swanick EJ, LaCamera F, Marriott HJ. Morphologic features of right ventricular ectopic beats. Am J Cardiol 1972;30:888.
14. Gozensky C, Thorne D. Rabbit ears: an aid in distinguishing ventricular ectopy from aberration. Heart Lung 1974;3:634.
15. Wellens HJ, et al. Medical treatment of ventricular tachycardia: considerations in the selection of patients for surgical treatment. Am J Cardiol 1982;49:186.
16. Gulamhusein S, et al. Electrocardiographic criteria for differentiating aberrancy and ventricular extrasystole in chronic atrial fibrillation: validation by intracardiac recordings. J Electrocardiol 1985;18:41.
17. Kindwall KE, Brown J, Josephson M. Electrocardiographic criteria for ventricular tachycardia in wide complex left bundle branch morphology tachycardias. Am J Cardiol 1988;61:1279.
18. Akhtar M, et al. Wide QRS complex tachycardia: reappraisal of a common clinical problem. Ann Intern Med 1988;109:905.
19. Brugada P, et al. A new approach to the differential diagnosis of a regular tachycardia with a wide QRS complex. Circulation 1991;83:1649.
20. Antunes E, et al. The differential diagnosis of a regular tachycardia with a wide QRS complex on the 12-lead ECG. PACE 1994;17:1515.

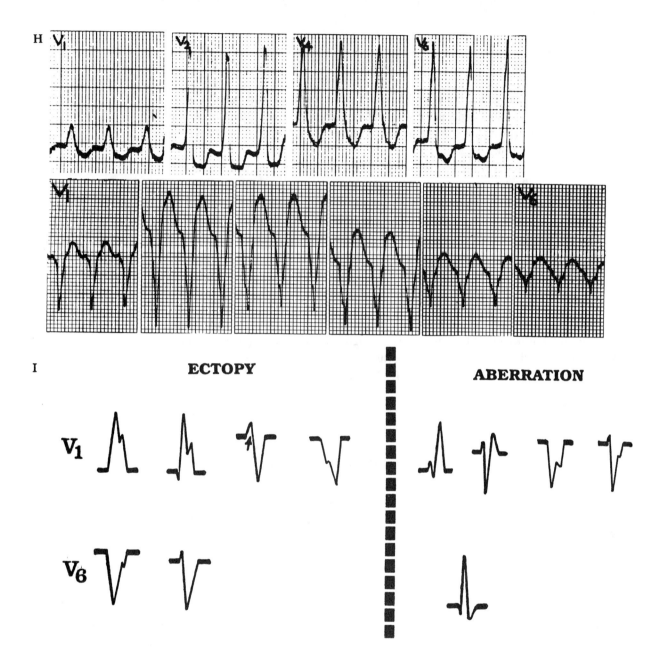

FIG. 11. *(continued)*

H – Concordance: **Upper panel** illustrates positive concordance; **lower panel,** negative concordance.

I – Important QRS shapes strongly suggesting ectopy or aberration.

LOOK-ALIKE QRS COMPLEXES

I have often seen others assume that a QRS complex, because it looks rather similar to those around it, has the same origin as the surrounding QRS complexes. Often this is not so. The simplest way to avoid this booby trap is to remember the aphorism: You cannot establish sameness from a single lead.

Figures 12-A and B display two examples of premature QRS complexes in lead H5 (Holter recording with electrode at V5 position) that would almost certainly be accepted without question as supraventricular because they look relatively narrow and so similar to the flanking conducted beats. But a glance at the simultaneously recorded lead H1 clearly shows that the beats in question are quite different and may well be ectopic ventricular.

Figure 12-C shows atrial fibrillation. In lead H5 it is impossible to recognize the grossly aberrant beats that are so obvious in lead H1.

Figure 12-D shows a beautiful example of sinus rhythm with LBBB interrupted by a couple of RV end-diastolic extrasystoles. At first glance, the strip of lead H1 appears to be all LBBB, but the third and fifth beats in the simultaneous lead H5 testify to their marked difference. On closer inspection of H1, these beats are slightly premature and the downstroke is more gradual than that of the LBBB beats (a clue to right ventricular ectopy—see #11); and of course the simultaneous complexes in H5 betray the typical concordant negativity of RV ectopy.

Figure 12-E shows atrial fibrillation with a slow ventricular response and then takeover by an idioventricular rhythm from the LV (concordant positivity). The last three beats in H5 are so similar that one would not suspect that the first of the three represented an intermediate form (probably a fusion beat between fibrillatory and idioventricular impulses); but when looking at this beat in H1, the intermediate form is evident.

Finally, Figure 12-F shows VPBs in three leads. In V5, the VPBs are virtually identical with the flanking conducted beats, whereas in leads 3 and V3 they are grossly dissimilar. The leads are not simultaneous, and therefore one cannot be absolutely certain that all the VPBs come from the same focus; but it would be unreasonable to conclude otherwise because (1) in long strips of each lead, the morphology of the ectopic beats was unchanging; and (2) the coupling interval is the same in all three of the displayed leads.

In the next five figures, which are from Holter recordings, H1 5 Holter lead with the electrode at the V1 position, and H5 5 Holter lead with the electrode at the V5 position.

FIG. 12.

A – Simultaneous Holter leads. In lead H5, the fourth beat looks enough like the flanking sinus beats that one is likely to call it supraventricular; but lead H1 shows that this beat has a very different configuration and may be ectopic ventricular.

B – Simultaneous Holter leads. In lead H5, the second, fourth, and sixth beats look sufficiently like the sinus beats to be called supraventricular; but H1 indicates that these three beats have a different contour and are probably ectopic ventricular.

C – Simultaneous Holter leads during atrial fibrillation. All the beats in H5 look remarkably similar and it is impossible to recognize the gross RBBB aberration that H1 reveals in second and fifth beats.

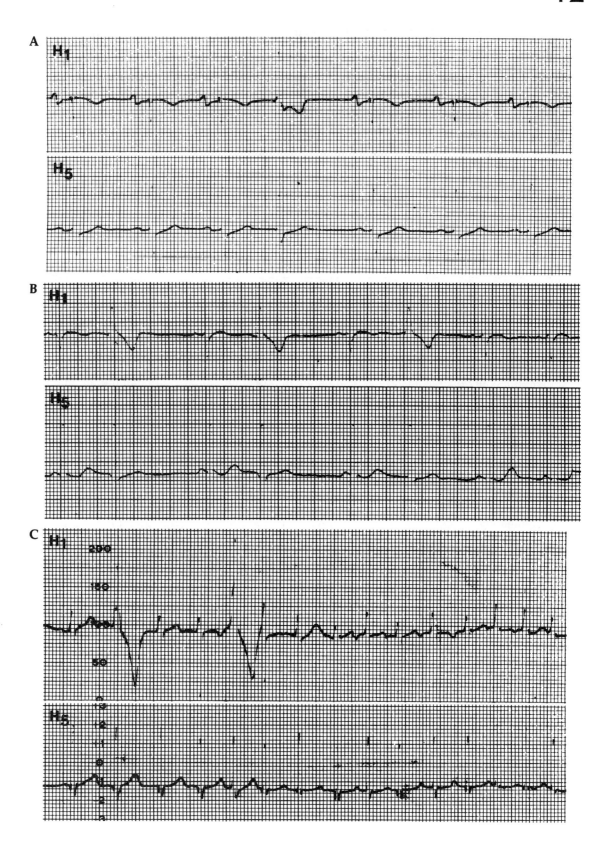

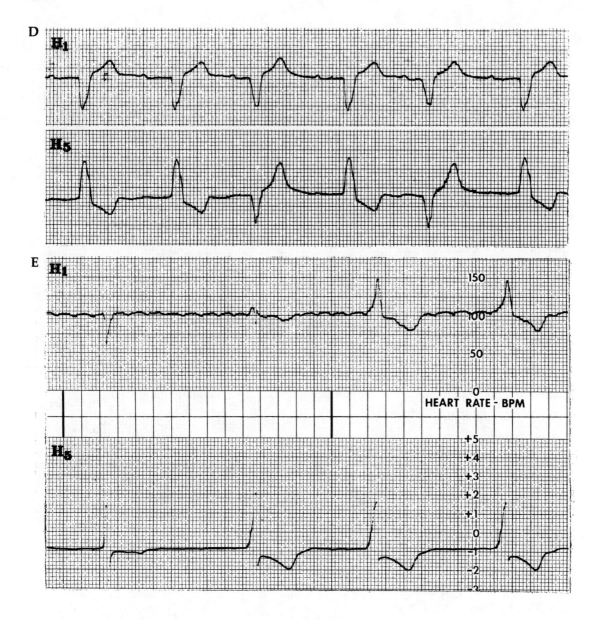

FIG. 12. *(continued)*

D – Simultaneous Holter leads. Superficial inspection of lead H1 gives one the impression that all beats are conducted with LBBB. Closer inspection spots the shorter P-R intervals of third and fifth beats. Lead H5 indicates that these beats are of different origin and are probably end-diastolic ventricular extrasystoles. Closer observation of these two beats in H1 identifies the more gradual downstroke, which is typical of ventricular ectopy in a right chest lead (V1 or MCL1—see #11). These beats also show concordant negativity (see #11), which favors ventricular ectopy.

E – Simultaneous Holter leads during atrial fibrillation, with the beginning of a run of presumable ventricular escape (note positive concordance, see #11). From lead H5, one might assume that the second, third, and fourth beats are identical; but H1 shows that the second beat is a transitional form and is presumably a fusion beat.

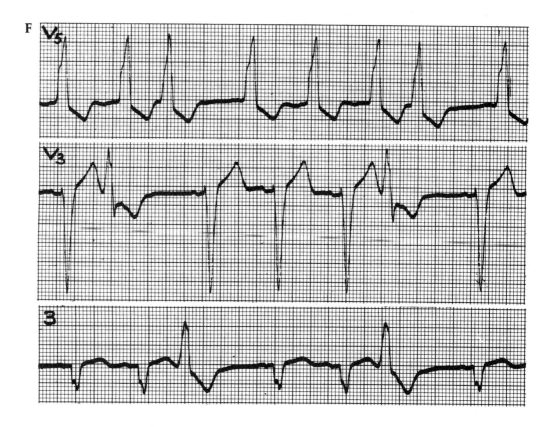

FIG. 12. *(continued)*

F – The three leads are not simultaneous, but it is reasonable to assume that all of the ventricular extrasystoles, with their identical coupling intervals, arise from the same focus. Note the close similarity of the premature beats to the conducted sinus beats in V5, whereas the dissimilarity in the other leads is striking.

13 P WAVES: ANTECEDENT BUT UNATTACHED

The two anomalous beats in Figure 13-A may be thought to be conducted with aberration because they are preceded by P waves. But inspection of the P-R intervals, and comparison with those of the conducted beats, promptly negates this notion—the P-R intervals of the anomalous beats being clearly too short for conduction. The shape of the left ventricular ectopic (top strip) is not helpful in the differential diagnosis, but the right ventricular ectopic (bottom strip) is typical in that there is slurring in the downstroke with nadir reached only after 0.08 s; a point in favor of ectopy rather than LBBB (see #11).

Because the P waves in Figure 13-A precede an early QRS, despite the fact that the P waves themselves are not premature, they are enveloped with an aura of prematurity and may be hastily mistaken for APBs with aberration. This is reminiscent of "number attraction," a grammatical ploy where, because the noun adjacent to the verb is plural, the verb is "sucked into" plurality even though its more remote subject is singular, e.g., "the supply of antiarrhythmics and other *drugs were* quickly used up" (should be "supply . . . *was*"). In a somewhat similar way, the premature QRS takes the preceding P wave under its wing and invests it with seeming prematurity.

In Figure 13-B, the bizarre QRS follows a premature P′ wave and might be mistaken for an APB with aberration. The clue again lies in the P-R interval. This premature P′ is simply one in the series of atrial bigeminy, and if you look at the P-R interval required for conduction of all the subsequent APBs (about 0.30 s), it is immediately obvious that the anomalous QRS cannot be a conducted beat. This is therefore a VPB precipitated by the lengthened ventricular cycle ("rule of bigeminy"—see #10) occasioned by the nonconducted APB at the beginning of the strip. This conclusion is again confirmed by the morphology of the anomalous beat, which has a sheer upstroke and a slurred downstroke typical of left ventricular ectopic beats (see #11).

In Figure 13-C, there are so many P waves (atrial tachycardia, rate 215/min) that it is impossible for a QRS not to be preceded by a P wave! However, the morphology—steep upstroke, slurred downstroke—identifies the anomalous beats as ectopic ventricular (see #11).

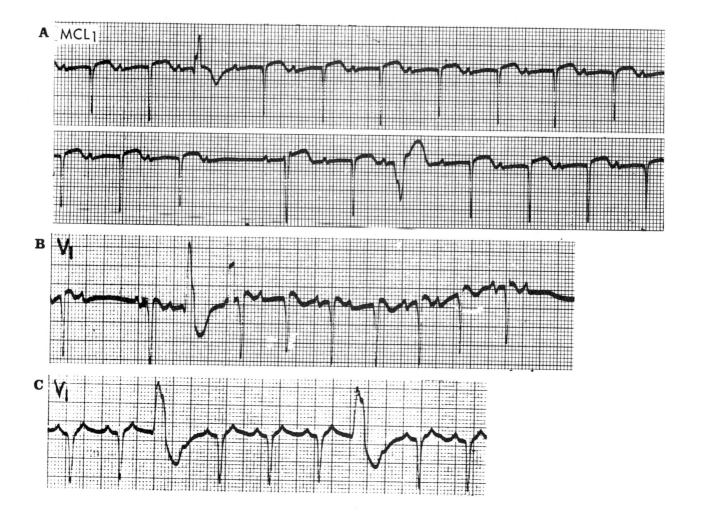

FIG. 13.

A – The two bizarre premature beats are VPBs (LV in the top and RV in the bottom strip); but, because they are preceded by P waves, a hasty and superficial appraisal might mistake them for APBs with aberration. Clearly they cannot be conducted because their P-R interval is considerably shorter than the demonstrably necessary longer P-R of the flanking beats. The shape of the wide QRS in the bottom strip is typical for RV (see #11).

The basic rhythm is sinus with slowly developing Wenckebach periods. The cycle of the dropped beat ends with a junctional escape beat with minor aberration.

B – Once again, because the bizarre beat is preceded by a P wave at a plausible interval, one might diagnose an APB with aberration; and indeed this time the P wave is ectopic and premature and represents the first in a series of APBs in bigeminal rhythm. But it is not conducted to produce the bizarre QRS—evidence for this is the fact that all the subsequent APBs require a much longer P-R interval for successful conduction. The shape of the anomalous QRS, with sheer upstroke and slurring on the downstroke, confirms its ectopic origin.

C – Atrial tachycardia, rate 215/min, with 2:1 conduction, interrupted by two left VPBs—note sheer upstroke with slurring on downstroke (taller left rabbit ear equivalent—see #11).

14 HAZARDS OF HOLTERING

This time, before reading the description, commit yourself to an interpretation of the three tracings.

To anyone suffering from the "P-preoccupation syndrome," the little bumps marching their way through the ventricular cycles in Figure 14-A are irresistible P waves and lead to the mistaken diagnosis of A-V dissociation. Closer scrutiny, however, reveals a very low but ever present sinus P wave in front of each QRS complex. "I only saw it because I was looking for it! (1)" And again, "Not invisible but unnoticed, Watson! You did not know where to look and so you missed all that was important (2)."

The rhythm is therefore normal sinus and the dissociated bumps happen to represent the QRS complexes of a previous patient in this improperly erased Holter tape! This is a not uncommon anomaly and almost invariably leads to misinterpretation.

Figure 14-B shows a similar situation, except that in this case the sinus P waves are prominent and unmistakable. The smaller, somewhat faster, blips are relics of a previous patient's QRSs.

Figure 14-C is another example of an incompletely erased tape. This time the previous QRS complexes have retained a more realistic ventricular morphology—they are inverted. However, when the tape was reused, it was not rewound and the second tracing was recorded on the tape in reverse!

REFERENCES

1. Sherlock Holmes in Silver Blaze.
2. Sherlock Holmes in A Case of Identity.

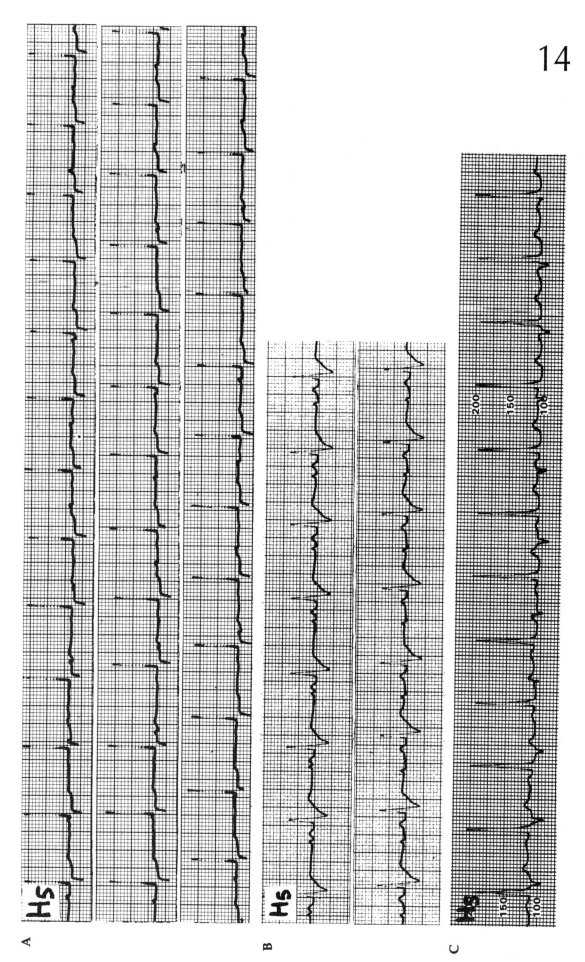

14

15 THE DISENGAGED ELECTRODE

Tracings like these (Figs. 15-A and B) have been published as periods of cardiac asystole. They are of course due to the temporary detachment of an electrode during the period of Holter monitoring . . . clearly an important distinction to make!

This form of artifact is readily recognized by the sequential waning, disappearance, and then waxing of the QRS complex—as electrode contact diminishes and then becomes reestablished.

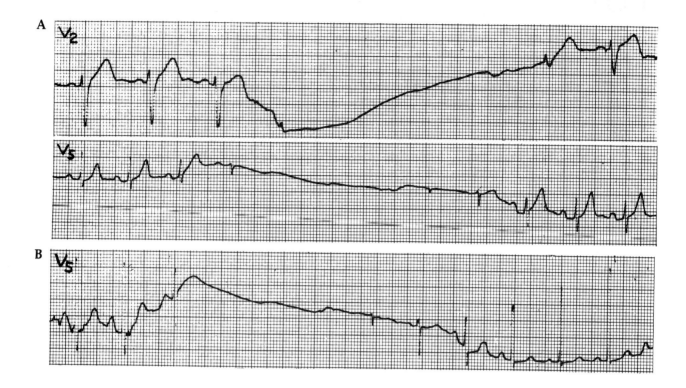

15

A

V_2

V_5

B

V_5

16 THE "TUP" PHENOMENON

Another simple booby-trap occurs when the T wave, U wave, and P wave, all having similar amplitudes, conspire to simulate an uneven baseline remarkably like that of atrial fibrillation (Figs. 16-A and B). The trap can be avoided by observing the regularity of the ventricular rhythm, by seeking and finding the hump of a P wave at a consistent, conductible interval in front of each QRS complex, and by observing the consistent sequence of the baseline undulations between the QRSs.

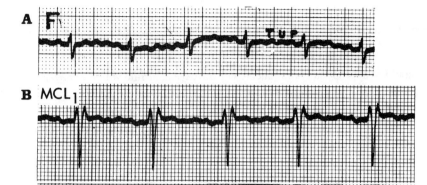

16

17 P-LIKE WAVES

This item could be appropriately introduced with the caveat: "Mind your P's; never mind your Q's!" The burden of this counsel is to be wary of things that look like P waves. This is particularly apposite when the P-like wave is close to the QRS complex: *it is often part of the QRS*. Figures 17-A to E present a variety of P-like waves that could easily deceive the hasty or unwary interpreter.

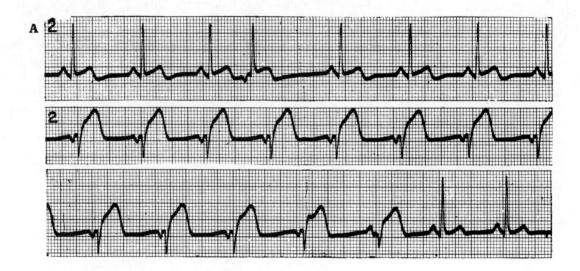

FIG. 17.

A – From a patient with acute inferior infarction (second and third strips are continuous). The top strip shows sinus rhythm interrupted by a single junctional premature beat, the retrograde P wave preceding the QRS at a short P-R interval. The second strip apparently shows the same retrograde P wave closely preceding a now inverted QRS complex; but, in fact, it is an accelerated idioventricular rhythm and the seeming P wave is part of the QRS complex. Proof of this resides in the fifth beat in the bottom strip. Judging by the P-R interval of the sinus rhythm in top and bottom strips, an interval of 0.14 s is required for normal conduction. If the inverted P-like wave were indeed a P wave, and the QRS began only with the second negative deflection, then the fifth beat in the bottom strip has an adequate P-R (0.15 s) for conduction. But there is no conduction. That is because the QRS begins with the small P-like wave and the actual P-R interval is only 0.05 s—hence no conduction.

   The mistake here could have been avoided by preoccupation with the QRS instead of the P wave (see principles of arrhythmic diagnosis in #1). The interpreter, observing the sudden reversal of polarity of the QRS, from predominantly upright in the top strip to entirely negative in the second strip, should focus his whole attention on the QRS and ignore P waves. The QRS inversion should immediately arouse suspicion and make him or her hesitant to diagnose two conducted rhythms with such disparate ventricular complexes. (Tracing courtesy of Dr. Gerard Church).

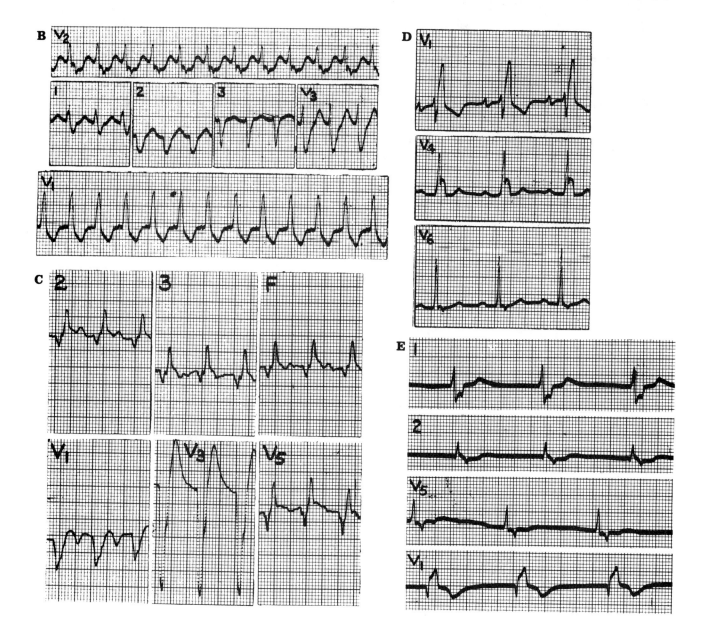

17

FIG. 17. *(continued)*

B – In this supraventricular tachycardia with RBBB, lead V3 documents the true width of the QRS complex. The rhythm strip of V2 looks like a narrow-QRS tachycardia with inverted P waves immediately following the QRS; whereas in V1, the first part of the QRS might be mistaken for antecedent atrial activity.

C – Here the Q waves in leads 2, 3, and a VF could easily be mistaken for the antecedent retrograde P waves of a junctional tachycardia. Leads V1 and V3, however, clearly document the full width of the QRS complex and demonstrate that the P-like waves in the inferior leads must be part of the QRS complex.

D – An example of RBBB in which the terminal S wave in V6 looks like an inverted retrograde P wave following a normally narrow QRS complex.

E – Another unmistakable RBBB pattern in leads 1 and V1. But in leads 2 and V5, the terminal part of the QRS looks like an inverted P wave. This illusion is enhanced by the fact that there are no P waves preceding the QRS complexes, presumably because the rhythm is junctional.

18 THE BIFID T WAVE

A fairly common trap is the young child's tracing whose bifid mid-precordial T waves—usually in V2 or V3—are mistaken for T-plus-P waves. Tracings such as that in Figure 18-A are often misdiagnosed as sinus or atrial tachycardia with 2:1 A-V block. Two further examples of bifid T waves are shown in Figures 18-B and C.

FIG. 18.

A – Sinus arrhythmia in an 8-year-old child. This should not be mistaken—as it has been—for atrial tachycardia with 2:1 block for two reasons: (1) the P-like fraction of the T wave is morphologically different from the P waves in front of each QRS and (2) it would be a most unusual atrial tachycardia to show such irregularity in the P-P intervals.

B – The three strips are continuous and are from another young child with sinus arrhythmia. Again, this should not be mistaken for atrial tachycardia with block for the same reasons as in Fig. 18-A.

C – Three precordial leads from an adult with LVH. In this case, the bifid T wave in V2, producing a P-like wave, is simply an intermediate form between the upright T to its right and inverted T to its left.

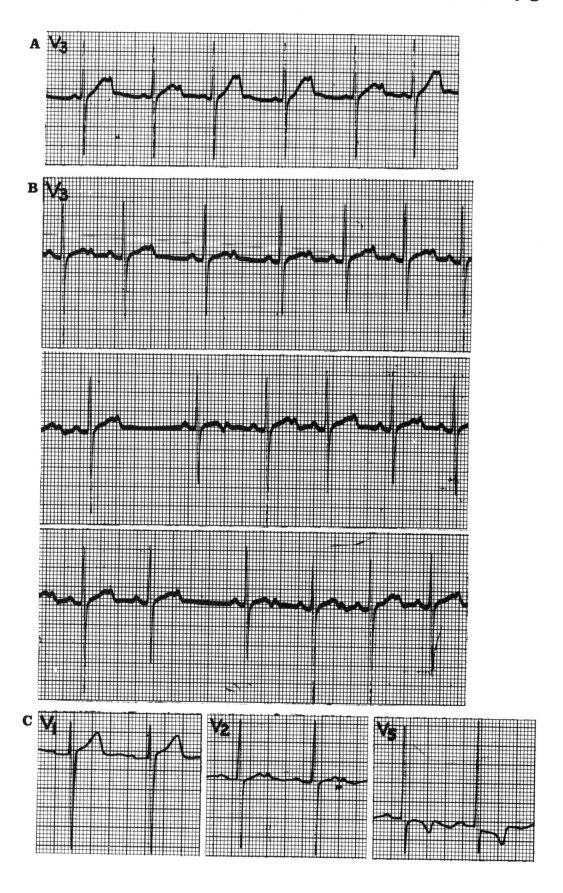

18

19   MASQUERADING U WAVES

Not only can part of the QRS complex and a peak of a bifid T wave be mistaken for P waves, but also the forgotten U wave may loom large enough to simulate atrial activity. Figure 19-A illustrates a junctional rhythm in which the U wave in V2 led to the mistaken diagnosis of sinus rhythm with first degree A-V block. Tracings such as those in Figure 19-B have often been mistaken for a bizarrely atypical manifestation of type I A-V block, or what French cardiologists called "floating P-R interval."

In both figures the mistake could be avoided by recognizing the fact that the wave in question is remarkably broad for a P wave; and in Figure 19-B, one can easily avoid the mistake by applying step 4 in arrhythmic diagnosis (see #1): establish relationships. If this precept is logically applied, it is immediately obvious that the wave in question bears a constant relationship to the antecedent T wave and not to the subsequent QRS. It therefore "belongs" to the preceding cycle and has nothing to do with the QRS that follows it.

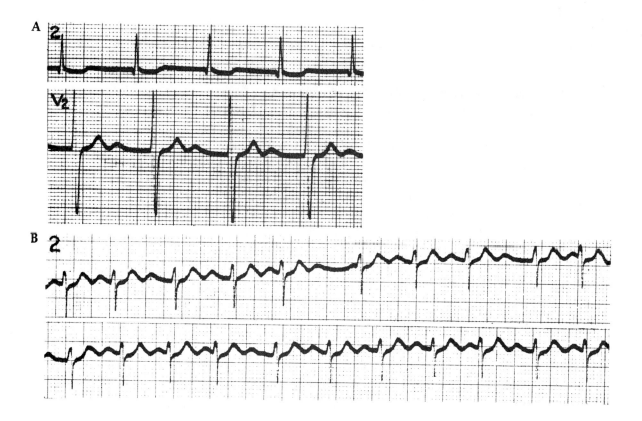

19

FIG. 19.

A – At a superficial glance, the rhythm in V2 could easily be mistaken for sinus with first degree A-V block. But if the supposed P waves are carefully evaluated, they are unusually—though not impossibly—wide for P waves. Their identity as U waves is clinched by looking at other leads (in this case, lead 2 shows no sign of atrial activity and establishes the diagnosis as accelerated junctional rhythm).

B – Atrial fibrillation in a patient receiving diuretics and with moderate hypokalemia. The prominent U waves, due to hypokalemia, superficially simulate P waves.

20 BROKEN REED

It is often taught that a VPB is followed by a fully compensatory pause, whereas a supraventricular premature beat is followed by a less than compensatory pause. This is a splendid general rule but there are so many exceptions to it that, to use the postectopic cycle as a helpful differential point, it is absolutely necessary to understand exactly why that general rule exists.

First of all, we need to agree on the usual way in which the postectopic cycle is evaluated. The common custom (Figs. 20-A and B) is to measure the two sinus cycles preceding the VPB (A-B) and compare them with the two cycles containing the VPB (B-C). If B-C equals A-B (Fig. 20-A), the postectopic cycle is said to be compensatory; if B-C is less than A-B (Fig. 20-B), the postectopic cycle is less than compensatory.

Now if nothing disturbs the regular discharge of the sinus node, B-C will equal the two sinus cycles A-B—because B-C in fact is two sinus cycles. On the other hand, if an APB comes along (Fig. 20-B), it will discharge the sinus node ahead of schedule and then, if the sinus wakes up again at the end of a normal cycle, beat C will be ahead of the original sinus schedule and the postectopic cycle will be less than compensatory. And so it should be clear that the postectopic cycle is usually dependent upon what is, or is not occurring, *in the atria*.

Now consider the exceptions. There are seven situations in which a VPB may be followed by a less-than-compensatory cycle:

1. The simplest and most obvious is when the VPB is interpolated; i.e., squeezed in between two consecutive sinus beats (Fig. 20-C).
2. If the VPB is premature enough, and sends its impulse backwards into the atria (an event that occurs in about 45% of VPBs [1]) so that it discharges the atria and sinus node ahead of the sinus schedule, then if the sinus node wakes up normally at the end of a sinus cycle, the postectopic cycle will be less than compensatory (Fig. 20-D).
3. If the VPB occurs against a background of sinus arrhythmia and happens to interrupt the accelerating phase, the two sinus cycles embracing the VPB will be shorter than the two previous cycles, and therefore the post-ectopic cycle will be measured as less than compensatory (Fig. 20-E).
4. If there should be simultaneous APB and VPB, it is the APB and not the VPB that determines when the next conductible sinus impulse will arise; and, provided the sinus wakes up normally after the APB, the postectopic cycle will be less than compensatory (Fig. 20-F).
5. If the VPB interrupts a developing Wenckebach period, the sinus beat following the interruption may enjoy better A-V conduction than the previous sinus impulse and therefore foreshorten the postectopic cycle (Fig. 20-G).
6. If the postectopic cycle ends with a junctional escape, it foreshortens the P-R interval and with it the postectopic ventricular cycle (Fig. 20-H). This of course is readily recognized if the shortened P-R is noticed; but if measurement is made by rote from the beginning of the QRS preceding the ectopic to the beginning of the QRS following the ectopic, the postectopic cycle will be measured as less than compensatory.
7. If the VPB interrupts a junctional rhythm, the returning junctional beat will usually end a cycle considerably less than compensatory (Fig. 20-I). This is because the ectopic impulse has retrogradely depolarized the AV junctional pacemaker before it was due to fire, and therefore the returning junctional beat is ahead of schedule.

NOT-SO-COMPENSATORY PAUSES!

THE USUAL SEQUENCE

The mechanisms of exceptions:

INTERPOLATION

EARLY VPB WITH RETROCONDUCTION

VPB DURING ACCELERATING PHASE OF SINUS ARRHYTHMIA

SIMULTANEOUS VPB AND APB

VPB INTERRUPTING TYPE I AV BLOCK

RETURNING BEAT AN ESCAPE BEAT

VPB INTERRUPTING JUNCTIONAL RHYTHM

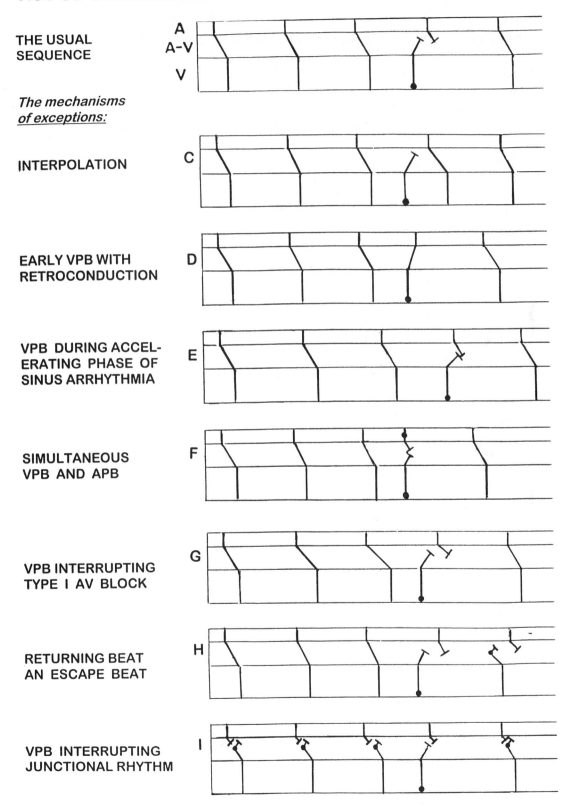

20

And then there are three situations in which supraventricular premature beats are followed by a fully compensatory pause:

1. Ectopic impulses tend to suppress pacemakers ("overdrive suppression"). Therefore, an APB may stun the sinus node so that it does not wake up until more than a normal sinus cycle has transpired. This SA nodal suppression may be sufficient to render the postectopic cycle fully compensatory (Fig. 20-J) or even longer.
2. If a junctional premature beat fails to be conducted retrogradely, the atrial rhythm continues uninterrupted and the postectopic cycle is fully compensatory (Fig. 20-K).
3. If instead of a single APB, there happens to be a pair (one of which is not evident because it is lost invisibly in the QRS complex, ST segment or T wave, and only the other atrial impulse is apparent), the ensuing cycle may measure as fully compensatory, or longer. In Figure 20-L, which illustrates this principle, the 4th beat is an APB conducted with prolonged P-R interval. The P′ wave of a second APB deforms the ST segment of this beat—if it had been slightly earlier, it would have been lost within the QRS complex.

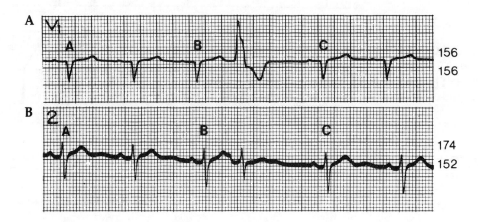

FIG. 20.

In all of the examples in this figure, the numbers at the right end of the tracing are in hundredths of a second; in each case, the upper number represents the interval A-B and the lower number B-C.

A – Typical findings with a ventricular extrasystole (BC = AB).

B – Typical findings with an atrial extrasystole (BC < AB).

C to I – Ventricular extrasystoles followed by less-than-compensatory pauses. **C.** Interpolated. **D.** With retrograde conduction (arrow). **E.** Interrupting the accelerating phase of sinus arrhythmia. **F.** With simultaneous atrial extrasystole. **G.** Interrupting developing Wenckebach. **H.** Postectopic cycle ending with junctional escape. **I.** Interrupting junctional rhythm.

J to L – Supraventricular extrasystoles followed by fully compensatory pauses. **J.** Atrial extrasystole with overdrive suppression of sinus pacemaker. **K.** Junctional extrasystole without retrograde conduction. **L.** Paired atrial extrasystoles.

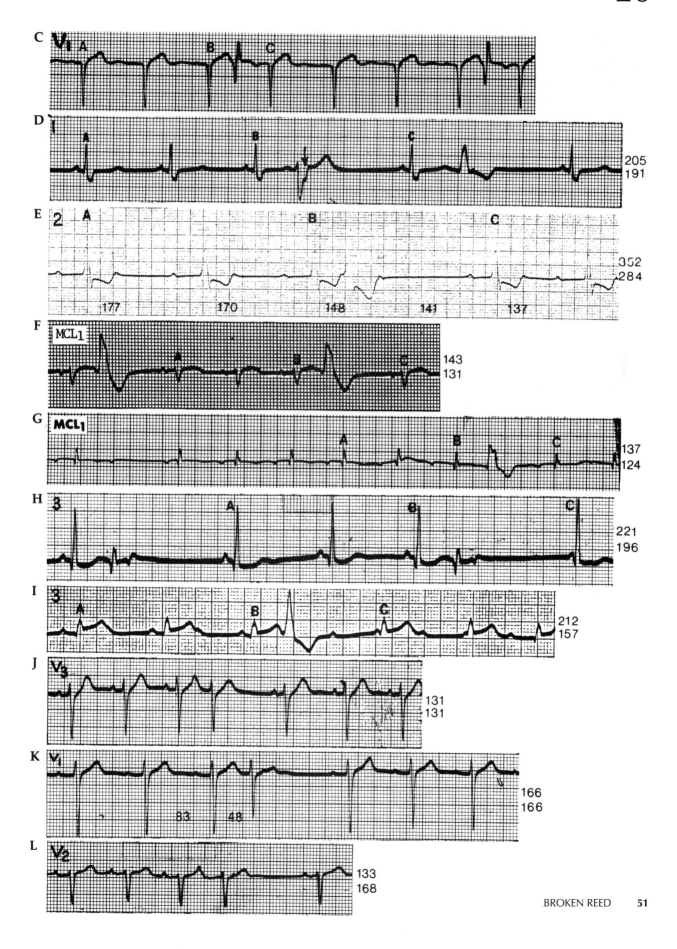

20

"One should always look for a possible alternative and provide against it (1)." It is diagnostically useful to keep in mind a number of pairs, knowing that when you see what you think is one of a pair you must exclude the other. "Unheavenly twins" is what I call these mutual mimics in the ECG. They may be difficult to differentiate, but they are well worth differentiating for one of two reasons: either because one is serious and the other relatively benign, or because the therapy of the two is quite different.

We have already encountered examples of such twins in #s 3, 10 and 11. Below is a listing of a dozen mutually imitative pairs.

20.1
TWELVE TWINS

WHENEVER YOU SEE WHAT MAY BE . . .	THINK OF AND EXCLUDE . . .	AND SEE . . .
a sinus pause	a nonconducted APB	#21
sinus bradycardia	nonconducted atrial bigeminy	#22
a VPB	an SVPB with aberration	#23
ventricular bigeminy	atrial bigeminy with aberration	#23
ventricular bigeminy complicating atrial flutter	atrial flutter with alternating 2:1 and 4:1 conduction with aberration of beats ending the shorter cycles	#3
an APB with aberration	fusion between simultaneous APB and VPB	#24
a ventricular ectopic beat during atrial fibrillation	Ashman's phenomenon	#10
ventricular tachycardia	supraventricular tachycardia with aberration	#11
progressive aberration	takeover by a ventricular rhythm via fusion beats	#25
aberration of the second beat in a row of rapid beats	VPB initiating reciprocating tachycardia	#26
junctional rhythm with reciprocal beating	dissociation between two junctional pacemakers	#27
second degree A-V block, type I or type II	concealed junctional extrasystoles	#28

REFERENCE

1. Sherlock Holmes in Black Peter.

PART 2
UNHEAVENLY TWINS

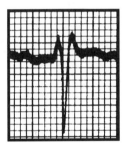

21 SINUS PAUSE VS. NONCONDUCTED APB

Whenever you see what looks like a sinus pause (Figs. 21-A and B), always be sure to exclude a nonconducted atrial premature beat (Figs. 21-C and D). A sinus pause may be evidence of a sick sinus, whereas a nonconducted atrial premature beat is usually of no consequence. To exclude a nonconducted APB, scan the baseline in the neighborhood of the preceding T wave for any sign of a blip or wrinkle, and carefully compare the T wave itself for any subtle change from previous and subsequent T waves.

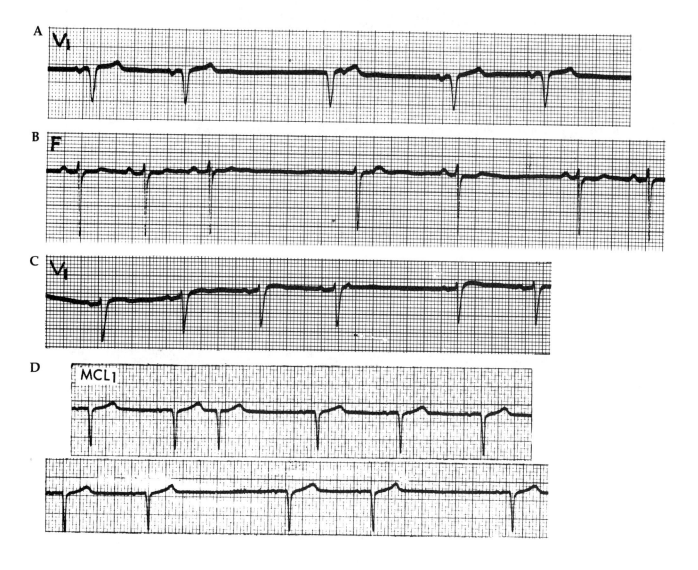

21

FIG. 21.

A – After two sinus beats, the next expected P wave fails to appear and the junction therefore escapes. A tardy P wave appears shortly after the junctional beat, and then sinus rhythm resumes.

B – After three sinus beats, the next expected P wave fails to appear and a junctional pacemaker therefore escapes. Shortly after the escape beat, and looking like a T wave, the P wave reappears and conducted sinus rhythm resumes. The last four P waves are deployed in pairs suggesting 3:2 sinus Wenckebachs (see #s 29 and 31).

C and D – After four sinus beats, a longer cycle results from a non-conducted APB (P' wave on ST segment of fourth sinus beat). Compare this easily observed P' wave with the difficulty encountered in Figure 21-D. After two sinus beats in the upper strip of Figure 21-D, there is a premature supraventricular beat. It is impossible to discern a premature P' wave and therefore impossible to tell whether it is atrial or junctional. In the bottom strip, there are two lengthened cycles. At the beginning of each cycle, the T waves are slightly, but definitely more pointed than any of the other T waves in the two strips. Clearly these are premature P' waves deforming the T waves, and measurement confirms that the premature beat in the upper strip was atrial rather than junctional because the long cycles in the lower strip (containing the recognizable premature P' waves) are identical with the cycle embracing the premature beat in the upper strip—where there must be an unrecognizable P' wave atop the T wave.

22 SINUS BRADYCARDIA VS. NONCONDUCTED ATRIAL BIGEMINY

The great imitator of sinus bradycardia is nonconducted atrial bigeminy, which may be easy (Fig. 22-A), difficult (Fig. 22-B) or impossible (Fig. 22-C) to spot. When it is undiagnosable in the tracing, it may sometimes be easily recognized at the bedside if cannon waves (resulting from atrial contraction while the tricuspid valve is still closed) are visible in the jugular pulse (Fig. 22-D).

Remember that cannon waves may be seen with both VPBs and APBs. How can they be distinguished at the bedside? If you are a good split-second timer, it's easy. With a ventricular extrasystole, the cannon wave occurs *after* the first sound (S1) of the premature beat, whereas the cannon wave occurs *before* the first sound of an atrial extrasystole (Fig. 22-E).

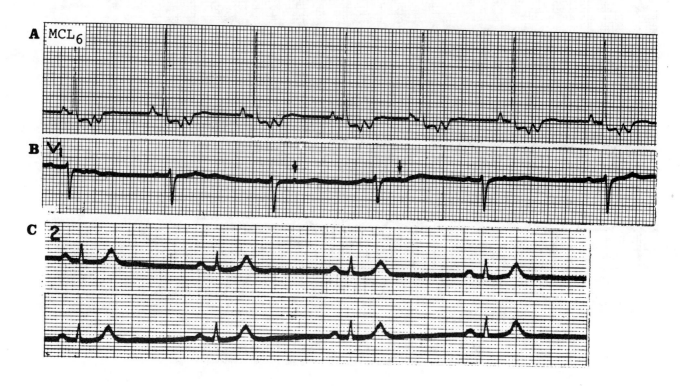

FIG. 22. NONCONDUCTED ATRIAL BIGEMINY

A – The P′ waves grossly deform the S-T segments and are inescapable.

B – The premature P′ waves produce tiny, easily missed, but definite bumps (arrows) on the S-T segments.

C – Nonconducted atrial bigeminy in a 10-year-old boy with a normal heart that is impossible to diagnose from the rhythm strip of lead 2, but is readily recognizable at the bedside by observation of the jugular veins (Fig. 22-D).

D – Note that the P′ waves, unrecognizable in lead 2, are clearly visible in V1, and that cannon waves (c) are conspicuous in the jugular pulse (jpt).

E – Diagrams that illustrate the mechanism and timing of cannon waves with VPBs and APBs.

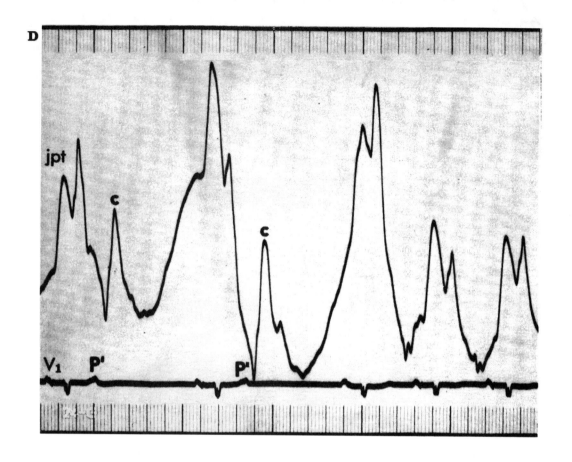

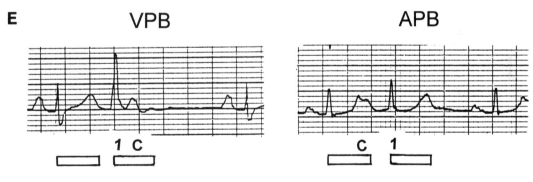

22

Key: Time of premature S1 = 1
Time of cannon wave = C
Approximate period with closed AV valves

23 VPB VS. APB WITH ABERRATION

It may be difficult to distinguish an APB with ventricular aberration (Fig. 23) from an ectopic ventricular beat. However, with careful scrutiny of three items, one can almost always discriminate between them. The three items to study are (a) preceding P′ wave, (b) QRS morphology, and (c) length of the postectopic cycle. Though any one of these can be misleading or at least unhelpful, if all three are carefully evaluated, few if any mistakes will be made.

PROBLEMS

The preceding P′ wave may be invisibly lost in the previous T wave; the morphology of the QRS in question may not be typical of either ectopy or aberration; and there are many exceptions to the compensatory pause rule (see #20).

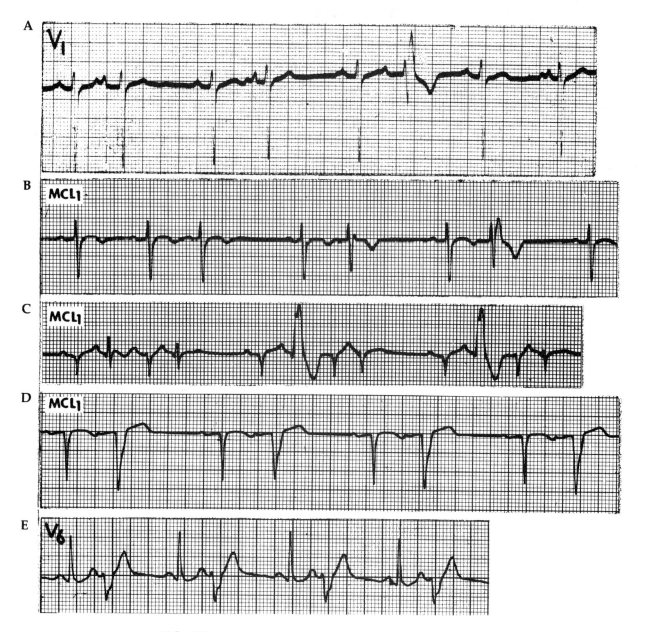

23

FIG. 23.

A – The sixth beat is an APB with RBBB aberration that is easily distinguished from a VPB by the rSR′ configuration, as well as the preceding premature P′ wave.

B – The seventh beat is an APB with RBBB aberration that is recognized mainly by the triphasic (RSR′) contour, the premature P′ wave being inconspicuous.

C – The sixth and tenth beats are APBs with aberration recognizable only from the preceding premature P′ wave; the QRS shape is entirely compatible with ventricular ectopy. Unfortunately, in these circumstances, one cannot always exclude the possibility of a simultaneous APB and VPB (see #24).

D – Atrial bigeminy with LBBB aberration. The preceding premature P′ waves are evident and the QRS contour is also helpful: there is a sheer downstroke with slurring on the upstroke favoring LBBB rather than RV ectopy (see #11).

E – Atrial bigeminy with bifascicular (RBBB + left anterior hemiblock) aberration; the rS pattern is imitative of LV ectopy.

24 APB WITH ABERRATION VS. FUSION BETWEEN APB AND VPB

When a premature P′ wave is followed by a distorted QRS complex, it is naturally diagnosed as an APB with ventricular aberration. But remember, it is always possible that you are dealing with simultaneous APB and VPB, with or without ventricular fusion. The importance of distinguishing is, of course, that the combination (APB + VPB) carries the significance of a ventricular rather than an atrial extrasystole.

In the top strip of Figure 24-A, each of the distorted QRSs is preceded by a premature P′ wave, and one's first thought is "APBs with aberration." Without the help of the lower strips there is no way to disprove that diagnosis. But in the middle strip, bizarre beats with identical coupling intervals have P′-R intervals that are too short for conduction; they are therefore presumably VPBs. And in the bottom strip, identical bizarre beats are not preceded by P′ waves. By inference, therefore, the beats in the top strip—despite their longer P-R intervals—are independent atrial and ventricular extrasystoles. Figure 24-B contains APBs (A), VPBs (V), and fusion (F) between simultaneous APB and VPB.

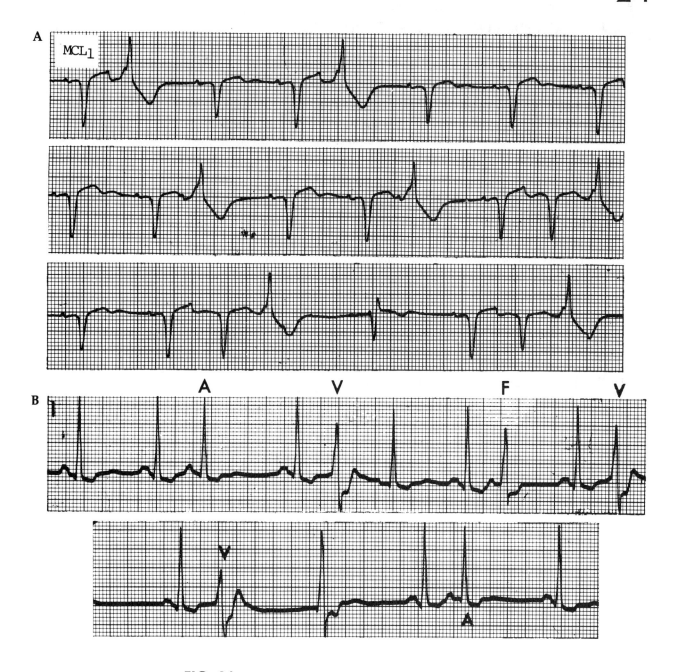

24

FIG. 24.

A – In the top strip, each bizarre QRS is preceded by a premature P wave at a conductible interval and the diagnosis of APB with RBBB aberration is naturally made. But in the middle strip, identical anomalous QRSs are preceded by premature P waves at an interval too short for conduction, and the last beat in the middle strip and both anomalous beats in the bottom strip are not preceded by any P wave. The anomalous beats in all three strips, therefore, are presumably ectopic ventricular. The diagnosis is further corroborated by the fact that all seven anomalous beats have identical coupling intervals.

B – The beat labeled F, consisting of a premature P wave followed by a distorted QRS, might at first be thought to be an APB with aberration, but the patient has both APBs (A) and VPBs (V). The distorted QRS of beat F has exactly the same coupling interval as beat V and somewhat resembles it; beat F is therefore more likely the result of fusion between a simultaneous APB and VPB.

25 THE WIDENING QRS: PROGRESSIVE ABERRATION VS. ECTOPIC TAKEOVER

There are three situations that produce a progressively lengthening QRS interval. The least common of these is the "concertina effect" in someone with WPW syndrome (Fig. 25-E). This is usually easy to recognize as the delta waves in successive beats become more and more prominent at the expense of the P-R intervals.

A problem, however, arises in distinguishing between the progressive development of ventricular aberration and takeover by an ectopic ventricular rhythm. The differentiation is easy if one remembers that it is impossible for an ectopic ventricular pacemaker to gain control without shortening the P-R interval. Thus, Figures 25-B and D display progressively shortening P-R intervals and are therefore examples of accelerated idioventricular rhythm taking over from the sinus rhythm via a run of fusion beats. On the other hand, as aberration progressively develops (Figs. 25-A and C), there is no reason whatever for the P-R interval to shorten, and so it remains constant.

In fact, the P-R interval may even gradually lengthen if the situation is complicated by type I A-V block. This may occur if the cause of the developing aberration is an accelerating sinus rhythm, which will automatically produce progressive shortening of the R-P interval and, since R-P/P-R reciprocity is the hallmark of type I block (see #30), the P-R interval will progressively lengthen as the rhythm accelerates.

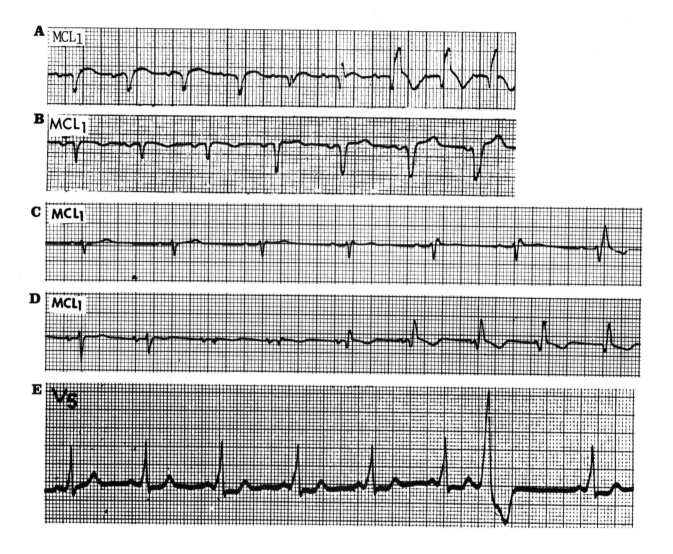

25

FIG. 25.

A and C – Two examples of sinus rhythm in which the QRS widens with each successive beat because of the progressive development of RBBB aberration. Note that the P-R interval remains constant.

B and D – Two examples of an accelerated idioventricular rhythm taking over from a slightly slower sinus rhythm via a succession of fusion beats. The QRS progressively widens as the contribution from the ectopic focus increases. After the first one or two fusion beats, note the inevitable shortening of the P-R intervals with each successive beat.

E – In the first six beats, the QRS complexes progressively widen at the expense of P-R intervals—the so-called "concertina" effect in the WPW syndrome. The seventh beat is a VPB.

26 WHEN ONLY THE SECOND-IN-A-ROW OF RAPID BEATS IS ANOMALOUS . . .

The refractory period of all parts of the ventricular conduction system—from the A-V node to the Purkinje network—is proportional to the preceding ventricular cycle, i.e., to the prevailing rate. Therefore, if you wish to encourage the development of block, the thing to do is to contrive to have a long cycle (which will lengthen the ensuing refractory period) followed by a shorter cycle (which will increase the likelihood of the next conducted beat encroaching upon the lengthened refractory period). Thus, depending upon which fascicle is most vulnerable, first degree A-V block, a dropped beat, or BBB is likely to develop. When the result is BBB, it is called ventricular aberration. A favored context, therefore, for the development of aberration is in the second beat in a row of rapid beats—by definition, such a beat will end a short cycle preceded by a relatively longer cycle. Thus, whenever one sees a burst of rapid beats in which only the second is anomalous (as in Figs. 26 A–D), one should always think of aberration.

Unfortunately, this phenomenon has a twin which may look identical to, and be indistinguishable from, a ventricular extrasystole that initiates a reentrant or circus-movement tachycardia. As is often the case when the distinction between ectopy and aberration must be made, one may have to rely upon morphologic and other clues such as those described in #11. In Figure 26-A, the diagnosis is almost certainly aberration because the anomalous beat is preceded by a premature P wave and the QRS has a forme fruste rsR'. In Figures 26-B and C, the morphology of the anomalous QRS is not helpful, but in each case there is a preceding P wave and the diagnosis again is presumably aberration. In Figure 26-D, morphology in lead 2 is of no help. The anomalous beat is preceded by a P wave but, judging by the needed P-R interval in the preceding conducted beats, the P-R interval is impossibly short for conduction and therefore the more likely diagnosis is a ventricular extrasystole initiating a reentrant tachycardia (see laddergram).

FIG. 26. ONLY THE SECOND BEAT IN RUN OF RAPID BEATS IS ANOMALOUS.

A to C – Examples of APBs conducted with RBBB aberration and initiating atrial tachycardia. A and C also each contain an isolated APB with aberration. In C, atrial activity is confirmed by positive bumps (arrows) on T waves preceding anomalous beats.

D – The strips are continuous. The fifth beat in the top strip is a ventricular extrasystole which initiates reentrant tachycardia.

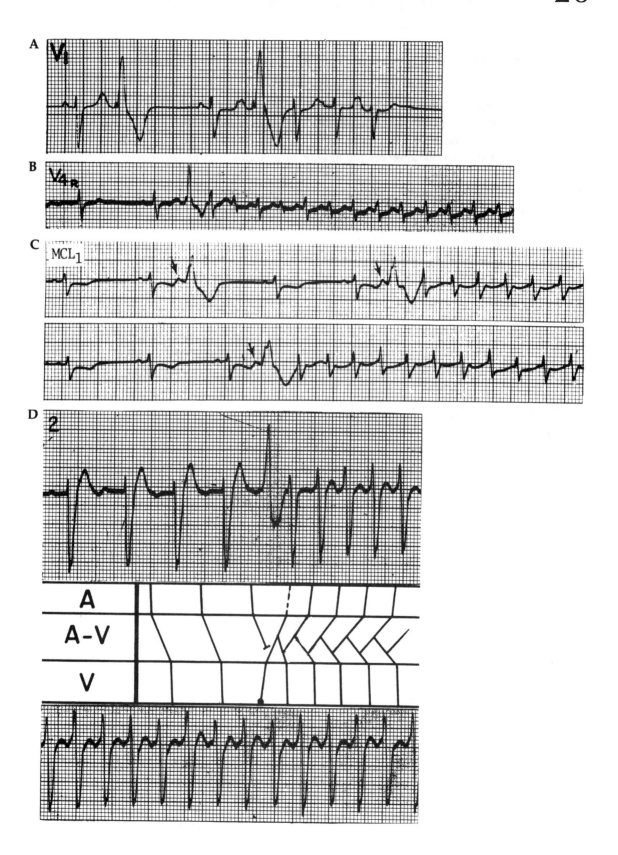

26

27 DISSOCIATION OR RECIPROCATION?

Another pair of mutual mimics is junctional rhythm with progressively lengthening retrograde conduction times ending with reciprocal beating, and A-V dissociation between two junctional pacemakers, the upper controlling only the atria (except for the occasional capture of the ventricles), and the lower controlling only the ventricles. Both of these mechanisms produce similar ECGs of retrograde P waves falling further and further beyond the QRS until, after a critical R-P interval, an early ventricular beat occurs.

How do you decide which is which? You measure the P-P intervals, and if the atrial rhythm is regular, you are probably dealing with A-V dissociation between two junctional pacemakers. But if the atrial rhythm is irregular, you are probably dealing with a junctional rhythm with reciprocal beating.

EXPLANATION

Most junctional rhythms are perfectly regular. Therefore, if the atria are under the control of an independent junctional pacemaker, the resulting retrograde P waves are usually regular (Fig. 27-A). But if the retrograde P waves are the result of progressively lengthening retrograde conduction, the P-P intervals will vary (Fig. 27-B)—just as the R-R interval changes in a developing anterograde A-V Wenckebach.

Now measure the P-P intervals in the figure and then study the subjacent laddergrams.

FIG. 27.

A – A-V dissociation between two junctional pacemakers, the upper pacemaker controlling the atria, and the lower controlling the ventricles, with occasional ventricular captures (C) by the upper pacemaker.

B – Junctional rhythm with progressive delay in retrograde conduction culminating in reciprocal beats (R).

Note the electrocardiographic similarity of the two sequences. The only difference in these particular examples is that the reciprocal sequence is completed in four beats whereas the dissociated junctional rhythms require seven beats. In beat one of each sequence, the retrograde P wave precedes the QRS; in beat two, the retrograde P has disappeared inside the QRS; in beat three, the retrograde P wave follows the QRS. Timing is such that in B, a reciprocal beat now occurs. In A, however, three more dissociated cycles are necessary before the upper pacemaker captures the ventricles and produces an early beat.

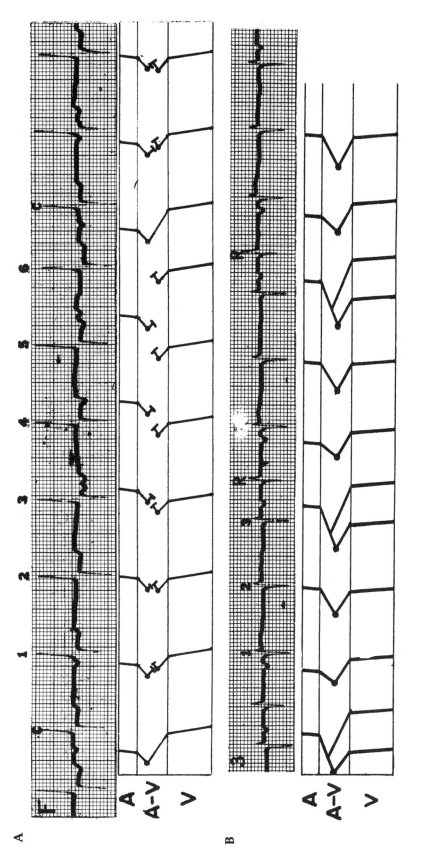

27

28 MIMICS OF A-V BLOCK CONCEALED JPBs

Concealed junctional extrasystoles are gremlins that inhabit the A-V junction and, on occasion, interfere with its conductive function. They can imitate both type I and type II A-V block (Fig. 28-A) and can produce sudden P-R lengthening (Fig. 28-B), or alternating P-R intervals (Fig. 28-C) (1). Although they can be proved only by intracardiac recordings, one can strongly suspect them in the following circumstances: If both type I and type II block appear to be present in the same tracing; if apparent type II block is associated with a normal QRS complex; or if there is sudden, unexplained lengthening of a P-R interval. Suspicion is greatly increased if any of these situations are seen in the company of manifest junctional premature beats elsewhere in the tracing (2). In fact, Langendorf accurately recognized concealed junctional extrasystoles as early as 1947 (3).

REFERENCES

1. Rosen KM, et al. Pseudo-A-V block secondary to premature nonpropagated His bundle depolarizations. Circulation 1970;2:367.
2. Langendorf R, Mehlman JS. Blocked (nonconducted) A-V nodal premature systoles imitating first and second degree A-V block. Am Heart J 1947;34:500.
3. Langendorf R. Alternation of A-V conduction times. Am Heart J 1958;55:181.

FIG. 28.

A – Each panel contains an ECG above and a corresponding His bundle recording below. In the **upper panel,** after two sinus beats with normal and constant P-R intervals (0.12 sec), the third sinus impulse is not conducted, therefore fulfilling the criteria for type II A-V block. The reason for the failure of conduction, however, is revealed in the His-bundle recording as an interfering His-bundle extrasystole (H'). In the **bottom panel,** the ECG contains a classical 3:2 Wenckebach period. The subjacent His-bundle recording demonstrates that lengthening of the second P-R interval is the result of a His extrasystole (first H'), and the "dropped beat" is due to a second premature His beat (second H'). (Reproduced with permission from the American Heart Association, Inc., from Rosen KM, et al. Pseudo-A-V block secondary to premature nonpropagated His-bundle depolarizations. Circulation 1970;42:367.)

B – In the **top strip,** there are two sudden, unexplained marked prolongations of the P-R interval. The **middle strip** shows similar P-R prolongation following what look like VPBs (x). Therefore, the picture here is one of interpolated VPBs with concealed retrograde conduction lengthening the postectopic P-R interval (see #37). But that does not explain the similar P-R lengthening in top strip. To explain the similar prolongations by a single mechanism requires that these seeming VPBs be something else; the only other possibility is that they are junctional premature beats with LBBB aberration. The **bottom strip** and its laddergram illustrate and diagram both mechanisms: the first junctional extrasystole enjoys neither anterograde nor retrograde conduction and is therefore "concealed," but it leaves the junction refractory and the next P-R interval is therefore prolonged. The second junctional beat similarly prolongs the next P-R interval, but, since it is conducted to the ventricles with LBBB aberration, is not "concealed." (Tracing courtesy of Dr. Leo Schamroth).

C – With every third beat being a concealed junctional extrasystole, alternating P-R intervals are produced (see laddergram). This mechanism of alternating P-R intervals was recognized by Langendorf long before His-bundle electrography became available (3).

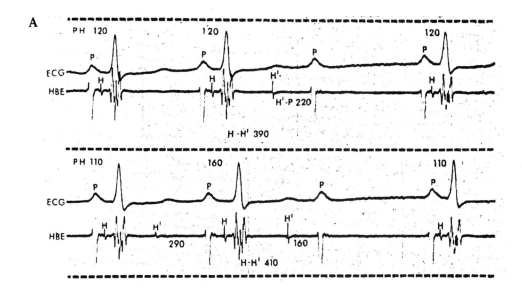

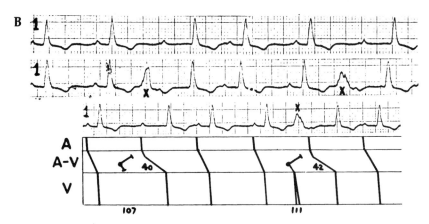

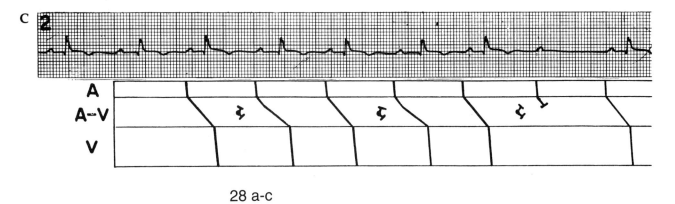

28 a-c

PART 3
MOSTLY BLOCKS

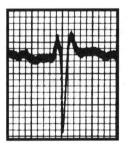

29 WENCKEBACH'S FOOTPRINTS

In 1899, Wenckebach described the type of A-V conduction that has since borne his name. The conduction pattern is typical of ailing A-V nodal behavior but is not peculiar to the A-V node. In fact, you may find the characteristics of Wenckebach-type conduction literally at any point in the heart where conduction occurs: out of the sinus node, out of an ectopic atrial focus, anywhere in the A-V junction, in a bundle branch, out of an ectopic ventricular focus, and even between a pacing electrode and the ventricular myocardium.

The characteristic behavior of Wenckebach-type conduction is that the conduction time grows longer and longer with each beat but by less and less, i.e., the increment decreases. Its features can be best understood by referring to a typical A-V Wenckebach period (Fig. 29-A) in which the progressively lengthening conduction time (P-R interval) is plainly visible.

If you look at the laddergram in Figure 29-A, you can see that the ventricular cycle is composed of the sinus cycle plus the increase (increment) in the P-R interval (75 + 10 = 85; 75 + 4 = 79). Because the increment decreases (from 10 to 4), the ventricular cycle proportionately decreases (from 85 to 79). The cycle of the dropped beat begins with the longest P-R interval and ends with the shortest P-R interval, and so it contains, not an increment, but a decrement. Therefore, the long cycle of the dropped beat is less than twice the shortest ventricular cycle.

The following summarizes the three "footprints" of Wenckebach conduction: (1) beats in small groups ("group beating"), especially pairs; (2) progressive shortening of the receiving chambers' cycle; and (3) the longest cycle is less than twice the shortest cycle (thanks to the dropped beat).

These characteristic features are usually present up to a ratio of 4:3. But if the Wenckebach period is longer (5:4, 6:5, 7:6, etc.), there is often an atypical feature—the commonest of which is paradoxical lengthening of the final P-R interval, as in Figure 30-A.

If we understand the structure of the Wenckebach phenomenon, we can recognize it without benefit of P-R intervals, and analogous conduction can be inferred in other sites. Figure 29-B is another A-V Wenckebach that we recognize, not by its lengthening P-R intervals, but by the immediate recognition of group beating and the fact that each group is preceded by a P wave at about the same prolonged P-R interval. It doesn't faze us when we cannot see the other P waves–from the footprints we can know what is going on.

These same footprints enable us to infer Wenckebach conduction at other sites: Figure 29-C shows a Wenckebach out of the sinus node; Figure 29-D illustrates one out of an ectopic atrial pacemaker; Figure 29-E illustrates one below the A-V junctional pacemaker; and Figure 29-F shows one out of a ventricular focus—all recognized by the typical footprints.

FIG. 29.

A – A 4:3 A-V Wenckebach period (same as Fig. 30-D). Note the shrinking P-R increment (10, 4), consequent shortening of the ventricular cycle (85, 79), and cycle of dropped beat (139) less than twice the shortest ventricular cycle (79).

B – Another A-V Wenckebach recognizable only by the footprints and because there is a P wave at a conductible and similar P-R interval preceding the first beat of each sequence.

C – A 4:3 exit Wenckebach out of the sinus node in an 8-year-old child with streptococcal tonsillitis (Tracing courtesy of Dr. Emory Hollar).

D – Atrial tachycardia with 3:1 A-V conduction and a 4:3 exit Wenckebach out of the ectopic atrial focus. (Tracing courtesy of Dr. Leo Schamroth).

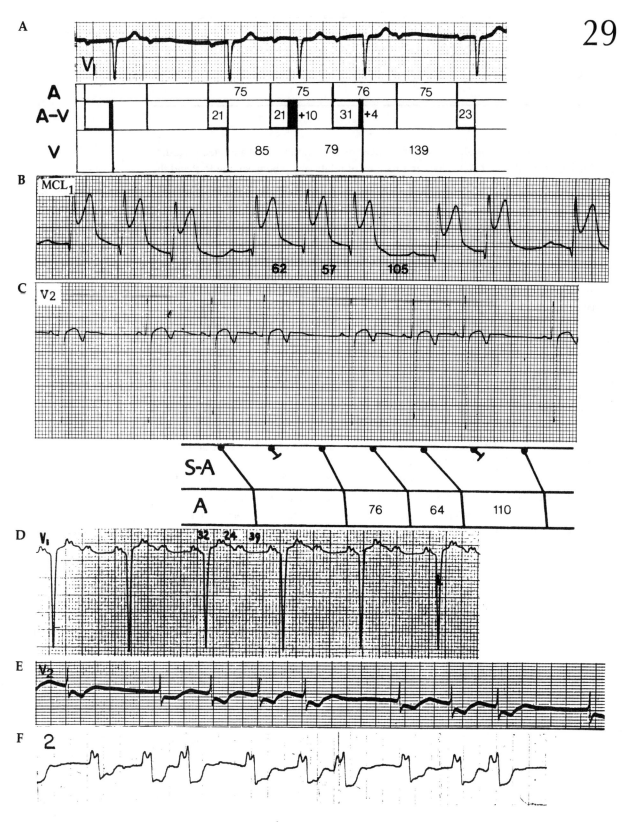

FIG. 29. *(continued)*

E – Accelerated junctional rhythm with 5:4 and 4:3 Wenckebach periods below the junctional pacemaker in a patient with digitalis intoxication and hypokalemia. The Wenckebach periods are typical except that the cycles of the dropped beats are longer than anticipated.

F – Ventricular tachycardia (or possibly junctional with LBBB) with 4:3 Wenckebach out of the ectopic focus.

30   R-P/P-R RECIPROCITY

Although it is there for all to see, few appear to have noticed that the electrocardiographic hallmark of type I A-V block is a reciprocal relationship between the R-P and the P-R intervals. "You see but you do not observe (1)!" The shorter the R-P interval, the longer the P-R interval and vice versa. Figures 30-A to C illustrate this relationship.

Look at the Wenckebach period in Figure 30-A and you can see that consecutive R-P/P-R relationships are as follows:

129/26, 59/33, 55/37, 49/40, and 45/48

The reciprocity is obvious and may be even more convincing if the relationship is seen to persist in reverse. So look at Figure 30-B in which, after three sinus beats with normal conduction, an APB is conducted with a much prolonged P-R interval (0.48 s). Following this, the next four R-P intervals become progressively longer whereupon each P-R interval adapts reciprocally to its antecedent R-P interval and progressively shortens—just the opposite to what happens in a Wenckebach period, but still having that same reciprocal relationship.

In Figure 30-C, the top strip shows normal A-V conduction with a P-R interval of 0.19 s. In the bottom strip, the initial sinus beat is followed by an APB which is conducted with a much prolonged P-R interval and subsequent sinus P waves therefore land near or on the T waves and suffer similar P-R prolongation.

Of course it is not the R-P interval itself that determines the P-R. The R-P is simply an indirect, but excellent, guide to the arrival time of the impulse at the sick region of the A-V node—the shorter the R-P interval, the earlier it arrives in the refractory period; the longer the R-P, the later it arrives. Figure 30-D diagrams this situation.

REFERENCE

1. Sherlock Holmes in Scandal in Bohemia.

FIG. 30. THREE TRACINGS ILLUSTRATING THE RECIPROCAL RELATIONSHIP BETWEEN R-P AND P-R INTERVALS IN TYPE I A-V BLOCK.

A – A 6:5 A-V Wenckebach period. The reciprocal relationship between R-P and P-R intervals is evident if you compare the R-P interval (recorded above strip) with the immediately succeeding P-R interval (recorded below strip). This Wenckebach is typical except for the disproportionate lengthening of the last P-R interval—probably the most common atypical finding.

B – The R-P/P-R reciprocity is maintained in reverse. After three sinus beats conducted with normal P-R intervals (0.19 s), an APB is conducted with a much prolonged P-R interval (0.48 s). In the next four (marked) cycles, sinus P waves land at progressively increasing R-P intervals and are therefore complemented by progressively decreasing P-R intervals (see table at right).

C – In the upper strip there is sinus rhythm with normal P-R intervals; after one sinus beat in bottom strip, an APB creates a shorter R-P interval and reciprocally lengthens the ensuing P-R interval to about 0.56 s. As a result, subsequent sinus P waves land near or on T waves and are conducted with similarly prolonged P-R intervals.

D – A classic 4:3 A-V Wenckebach (same as in Fig. 29-A). Consecutive P-R intervals are 21, 31, and 35. The diagram under the tracing is drawn to scale and its numbered impulses correspond with the respective P waves in the tracing. Dark stippling represents the absolute refractory period and lighter stippling the relative refractory period. Note that the interval from 1 to 2 represents a major retreat into the refractory period and therefore produces the larger increase in the P-R interval.

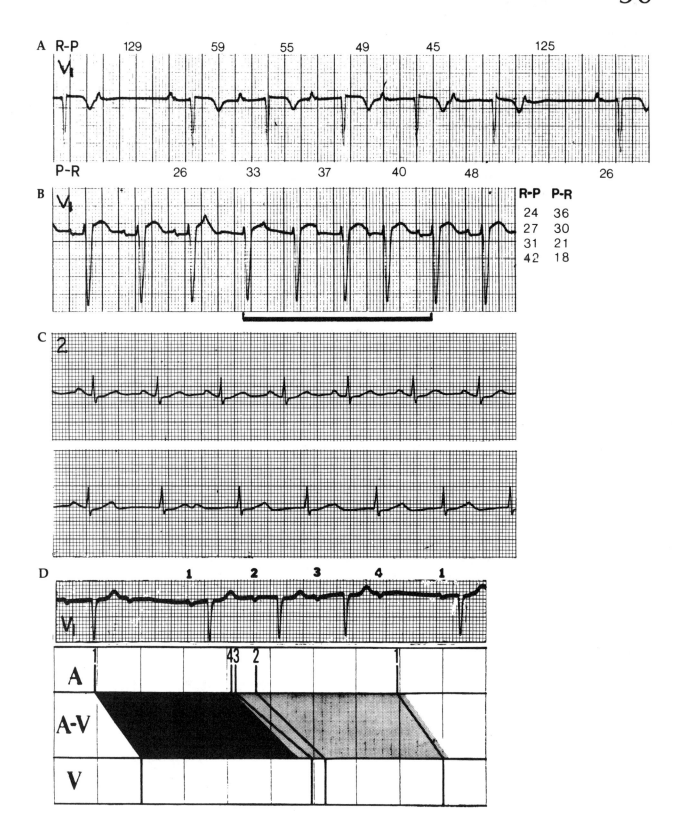

30

31 PAIRS GALORE

We have seen that group beating immediately suggests the Wenckebach phenomenon at work (#29). It is a moot question whether a "group" should include pairs. Do three clustered beats constitute the least number to form a "group?"

Regardless of semantics and whether or not a pair qualifies as the minimal "group," there is no question that of all deployments, pairing is highly suggestive of the Wenckebach. Figures 31-A to C, E and F present a selection of paired beats, all presumably due to the operation of 3:2 Wenckebach periods.

Of course, on rare occasions you will encounter type II A-V block in a 3:2 ratio producing paired ventricular beats (Fig. 31-D). When there are no P-R intervals to observe, you can tell the difference between a type I and a type II mechanism by comparing the length of the shorter cycle with that of the longer cycle. In type I block, the longer cycle is less than twice the shorter cycle, while in type II block (provided the basic rhythm is regular), the longer cycle is exactly twice the shorter cycle. In Figures 31-A to C, E and F, the longer cycle is less than twice the shorter—testifying to type I (Wenckebach) conduction.

FIG. 31. A PLETHORA OF PAIRS

A – A 3:2 Wenckebach out of the sinus node.

B – A 3:2 Wenckebach out of the atrial flutter focus. There is also a more gradual A-V Wenckebach at a level below the 2:1 "filter" (see laddergram).

C – A 3:2 A-V Wenckebach.

D – 3:2 type II A-V block. Note the normal P-R intervals and LBBB.

E – An accelerated junctional rhythm with 3:2 Wenckebach below the junctional pacemaker (see laddergram—from the same patient as Fig. 29-E).

F – RV tachycardia with 3:2 Wenckebach out of the ectopic ventricular focus (see laddergram; e = ectopic focus). There is also a thwarted retrograde Wenckebach to the atria—R-P intervals are lengthening (arrows indicate retrograde P waves)—but the potential retrograde Wenckebach is interrupted by the pause produced by the dropped ventricular beat.

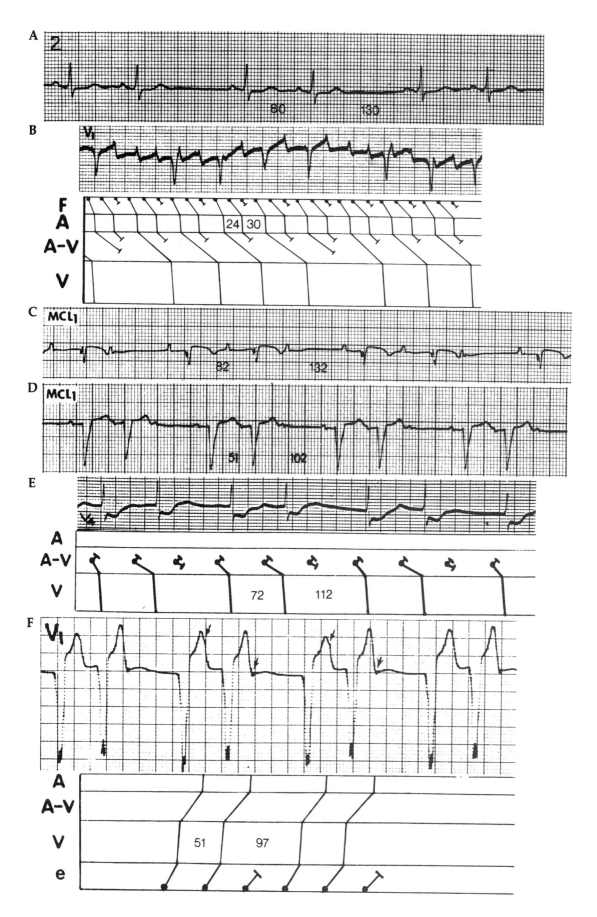

31

32 "OVER THE TOP"

Because of an illusion created when events occurring at multiple levels in the heart are recorded on two-dimensional paper, a very natural occurrence can look to many observers like an impossibility. If you study Figure 32, all the necessary evidence for diagnosing repeated Wenckebach periods can be seen: group beating, the longest cycles are less than twice that of the shortest cycles, and within each group, the first cycle is usually longer than the second. Thus, all the "footprints" are in place (see #29) and there is an obvious progressive lengthening of the P-R interval in each group of beats. But the first and second P-R intervals in all groups are too short for conduction—especially in someone with type I A-V block. The presence of Wenckebach conduction, however, is incontrovertible; and one must therefore attribute each QRS not to the immediately preceding P wave, but to the one before that (see the laddergram). "When you have eliminated the impossible, whatever remains, however improbable, must be the truth!"(1)

Now consider the interpreter's dilemma. On the two-dimensional paper, it looks impossible for an atrial impulse to be conducted "over the top of" a QRS complex to the next QRS. But, if you think of it logically, it becomes clear that the intervening QRS is irrelevant. If the atria have a mandate to beat at a certain rate, they will beat at that rate. And when it is time for the atrial pacemaker to fire, the atria could care less whether the previous impulse has reached the ventricles or not. To see this fact clearly, look at the laddergram which separates levels in the heart in a way that the tracing itself cannot. And don't be concerned about a P-R interval of more than 0.60 s; P-R intervals can be much longer than this as you will see in #33.

This same patient, at slower atrial rates, conducted 1:1 with P-R intervals slightly longer than the R-R intervals (Figure 32 B).

REFERENCE

1. Sherlock Holmes in The Sign of Four.

FIG. 32.

A – The strips are continuous. Sinus tachycardia (rate 125/min) with 3:2, 4:3, and 5:4 Wenckebach periods in a patient with acute anteroseptal infarction. (Reproduced from Marriott HJ. Practical Electrocardiography. 8th ed. Baltimore: Williams & Wilkins, 1988).

B – The atrial rate is now only 95/min and 1:1 AV conduction results with P-R intervals consistently longer than the ventricular cycle (laddergrams).

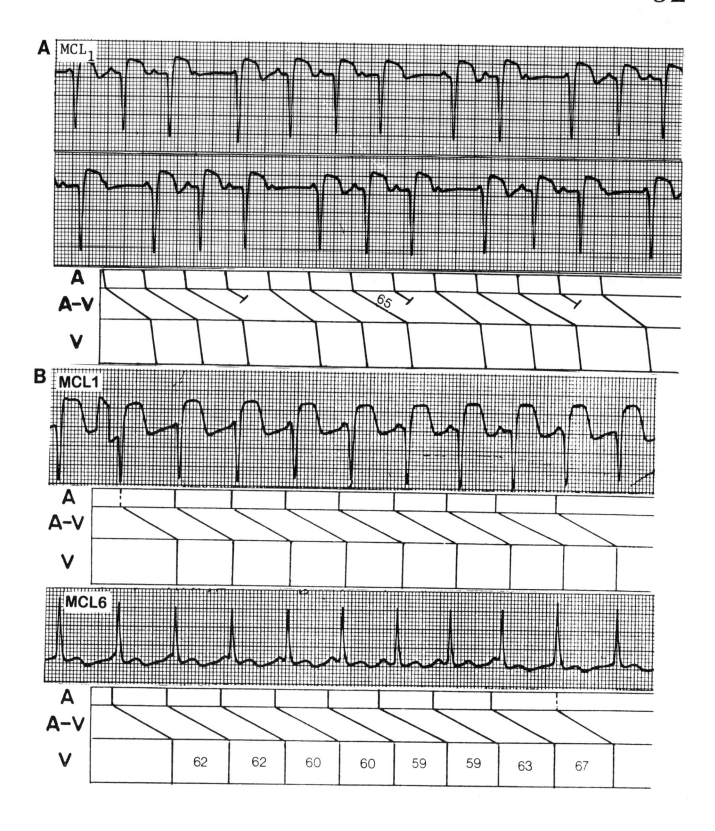

32

A MCL₁

A
A-V   65
V

B MCL1

A
A-V
V

MCL6

A
A-V
V   62   62   60   60   59   59   63   67

33 THE ELASTIC P-R

I have often been told by coronary care personnel that they were taught that you cannot have a conducting P-R interval longer than 0.40–0.50 s. The truth is that P-R intervals can attain twice such lengths, and that the longest P-R interval is usually found in the last conducted beat before the dropped beat of an A-V Wenckebach period. Figure 32 illustrated A-V Wenckebach periods in which the last conducted P-R interval measured 0.62–0.68 s. Figure 33-A illustrates the concluding cycles of a Wenckebach period in which the final P-R interval was 0.88 s. For P-R intervals over 1.0 s, see the published examples reproduced in Figure 33-B.

Another context in which the P-R interval may sometimes stretch to surprising lengths is in the conduction of an APB in patients with already much prolonged P-R intervals during sinus rhythm (1). Figure 33-C illustrates a patient whose P-R intervals during sinus rhythm were 0.81–0.85 s. With an APB, the interval stretched to 0.93 s. Figure 33-D, which certainly competes for the longest P-R interval published to date, presents a patient whose sinus P-R intervals were 0.94–0.96 s in whom an APB is conducted with a P-R interval of 1.10 s.

REFERENCE

1. Rusterholz AP, Marriott HJ. How long can the PR interval be? Am J Noninvas Cardiol. 1994;8:11.

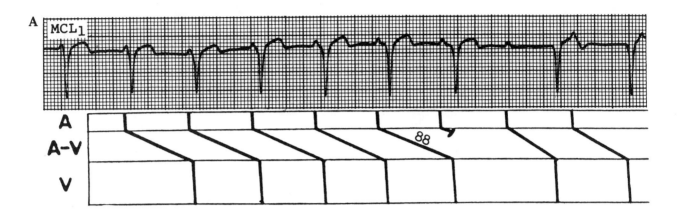

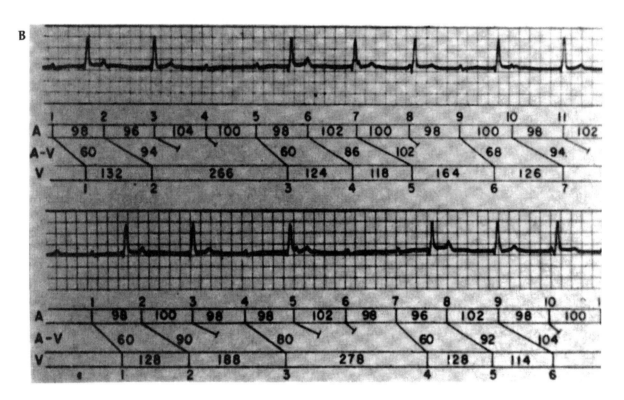

FIG. 33.

A – The last few cycles of a prolonged Wenckebach period in which the final P-R interval attains a length of 0.88 s.

B – An example of A-V Wenckebach periods in which the final P-R intervals reach 1.02 and 1.04 s. (I am unable to give appropriate credit for this illustration and here apologize to the copyright owner. I photographed the tracing several years ago and, despite a diligent search, have been unable to resurrect the original article in which it appeared. I believe it is from a publication by Alfred Pick and Richard Langendorf but cannot be sure. If any reader recognizes the source, I would deeply appreciate a communication).

33

FIG. 33 (*continued*)

C – Sinus rhythm with P-R intervals ranging from 0.81 to 0.85 s; an earlier atrial impulse requires 0.93 s for conduction.

D – Sinus rhythm with P-R intervals ranging from 0.94–0.96; an earlier impulse is conducted with a P-R interval of 1.10 s.

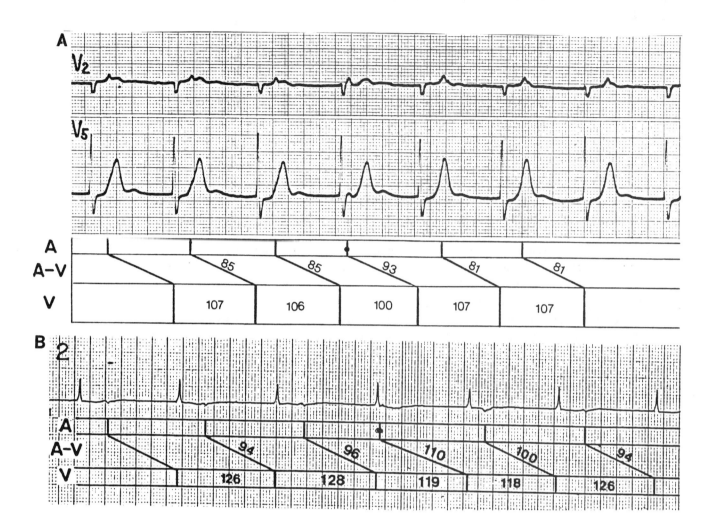

34 REVERENCE FOR RATIOS

For some unknown reason, there has been an almost universal tendency to equate the severity of A-V block with the A-V conduction ratio. This is particularly true of 2:1 conduction. Thus, respected authorities have stated that a 2:1 ratio makes the block high grade or advanced (1,2). It takes but a moment's thought, however, to realize that if you don't take the rate into consideration, the ratio is almost meaningless. If 2:1 conduction is present when the atrial rate is about 60/min (Fig. 34-A), it is bad news and indeed may justifiably be considered "high grade" A-V block; but, if the atrial rate is about 120/min (Fig. 34-B), 2:1 conduction may well be a blessing in disguise.

In the presence of atrial flutter with an atrial rate around 300/min (Fig. 34-C), a 2:1 conduction ratio should not even be called block because "block" implies abnormality, and a 2:1 ratio at an atrial rate of 300/min means only that the A-V node is doing its job in protecting the ventricles from phrenetic atrial behavior.

The two most important considerations in A-V block are not the A-V ratio, but (1) the level of the block (nodal or infranodal), and (2) the resulting ventricular rate. Just as BBB can be rate-dependent, so can ratios of A-V block. A patient who has 2:1 block at an atrial rate of 116/min, for example, may have only first degree block at an atrial rate of 100/min (Fig. 34-D). Anyone who can conduct every beat at a rate of 100/min certainly does not have high grade Λ-V block regardless of the ratio at a rate of 116/min.

MAXIM

Never assign significance to a conduction ratio while disregarding the prevailing rate.

REFERENCES

1. Josephson ME, Seides SF. Clinical cardiac electrophysiology: techniques and interpretations. Philadelphia: Lea & Febiger, 1979, p. 80.
2. WHO/ISC Task Force. Definition of terms related to cardiac rhythm. Am Heart J. 1978;95:796.

FIG. 34. EXAMPLES OF 2:1 A-V CONDUCTION AT VARIOUS RATES.

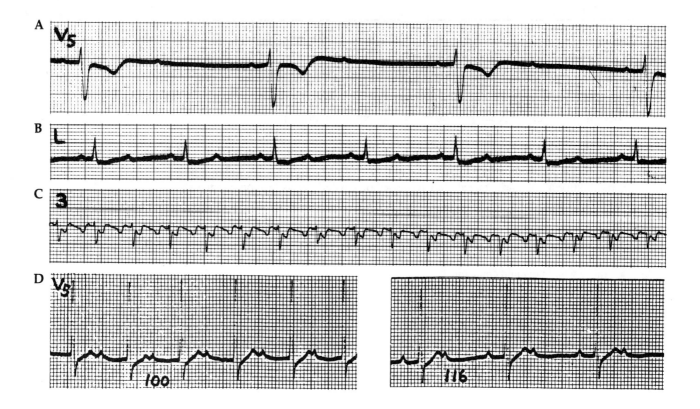

34

A – Atrial rate 54/min, ventricular 27/min.

B – Atrial rate 112/min, ventricular 56/min.

C – Atrial rate 280/min, ventricular 140/min.

D – Patient with 2:1 A-V conduction at atrial rate of 116/min has 1:1 conduction with only first degree A-V block at 100/min.

35 TWO-TO-ONE CHAOS

RIDDLE:

Q: Why is 2:1 A-V block like a split infinitive?
A: Because the English-speaking world adopts five positions for each.

At first, there is no obvious connection between the often desirable, but much maligned grammatical construction, the split infinitive and 2:1 A-V block. However, when I hear that A-V ratio pronounced, I am immediately reminded of Fowler's classification of English-speakers according to their attitude toward the split infinitive (1). He divided them into:

- those who neither know nor care what a split infinitive is
- those who do not know, but care very much
- those who know and condemn
- those who know and approve
- those who know and distinguish

The reason Fowler's droll classification comes to mind is that cardiologists can be similarly divided into five categories according to their beliefs about 2:1 block, each of which is supported by respected authority. There are those who believe:

- that 2:1 block is high grade or advanced block (2,3)
- that 2:1 block is type II block (4)
- that 2:1 block is neither type I nor type II block, but a genre all its own (5)
- that 2:1 block may be either type I or type II block, but you cannot tell which it is (3)
- that 2:1 block may or may not be high grade, may be either type I or type II — but is much more often type I—and that you often *can* tell which it is (6)

It is, of course, members of the last category that best understand the nuances of A-V block.

One important by-product of studying 2:1 block is realizing the vital significance of rate: the faster the atrial rate, the less the significance of a 2:1 ratio. Yet it has been common practice to lump all 2:1 blocks together as though the ratio alone determined the severity. A moment's reflection, however, tells us that 2:1 block at a rate of 130/min does not have the same significance as 2:1 block at a rate of 65/min (see #34).

Figure 35-A shows carotid sinus stimulation "curing" 2:1 A-V block—not by improving conduction, but by slowing the atrial rate and thereby lengthening the R-P interval enough to permit 1:1 conduction.

REFERENCES

1. Fowler HW. A dictionary of modern English usage. Oxford: Oxford University Press, 1944, p. 558.
2. Josephson ME, Seides SF. Clinical cardiac electrophysiology: techniques and interpretations. Philadelphia: Lea & Febiger, 1979, p. 80.
3. WHO/ISC Task Force. Definition of terms related to cardiac rhythm. Am Heart J. 1978;95:796.

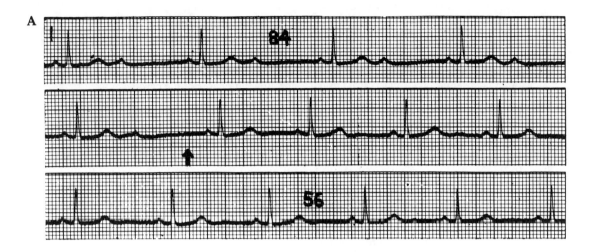

35

FIG. 35.

A – Strips are continuous. Carotid sinus stimulation applied at arrow slows the atrial rate from 84 to 56 and converts 2:1 A-V block to 1:1 conduction.

4. Escher DJ. Approach to conduction abnormalities in acute myocardial infarction, In Eliot RS, ed. Cardiac Emergencies, 2nd ed. Mt. Kisco: Futura Publishing, 1982, p. 313.
5. Barold SS. Modern Cardiac Pacing. Mt. Kisco: Futura Publishing, 1985, p. 974.
6. Zipes DP. Second-degree atrioventricular block. Circulation. 1979;60:465.

36 "COMPLETE" A-V BLOCK

To diagnose complete A-V block requires three criteria: (1) no conduction, despite (2) a slow enough ventricular rate, and (3) atrial impulses probing all phases of the cardiac cycle (Fig. 36-A).

What is "slow enough?" Most of us regard a rate of 45/min as a reasonable cutoff, although some require a rate less than 40/min (1,2). The reason for the stated criteria is simply this: to diagnose the ultimate in A-V block, there must be optimal opportunity for conduction. You can't diagnose absolute fidelity unless an optimal opportunity for infidelity presents itself and is resisted. By the same token, one cannot say that the block is absolute (complete) unless there is optimal opportunity for conduction. And the two things that make opportunity optimal are a slow enough ventricular rate and enough atrial impulses to test the A-V barrier in all phases of the cardiac cycle.

Although there may be argument as to the upper limit of the ventricular rate, there can be no argument that rates more than 50/min are beyond the reasonable limit. Yet innumerable authors appear to ignore the ventricular rate and base the diagnosis of complete block on two criteria: (1) evidence of some degree of A-V block and (2) absence of conduction (Fig. 36-B). Despite the fact that Langendorf and Pick (3) clearly demonstrated that minimal A-V block (first degree), when combined with a slightly accelerated ventricular rate, could inhibit all A-V conduction (Fig. 36-C), many respected authors have accepted the diagnosis of complete block with ventricular rates over 50/min (4), over 60/min (5,6), over 70/min (7), and even over 80/min (8). The relevant facts are that slight acceleration of the ventricular rate, combined with minimal block—whether the atrial rate is faster than the ventricular (Figs. 36-B and D) or the ventricular rate is faster than the atrial (Fig. 36-C)— is enough to prevent all conduction, at least for a time.

REFERENCES

1. Schamroth L. The disorders of cardiac rhythm. Oxford: Blackwell Scientific Publications, 1980, p. 540.
2. Pritchett EL. Office management of arrhythmias. Philadelphia: WB Saunders, 1982, p. 18.
3. Langendorf R, Pick A. Artificial pacing of the human heart: its contribution to the understanding of the arrhythmias. Am J Cardiol. 1971;28:516.
4. Chung EK. Principles of Cardiac Arrhythmias. 2nd ed. Baltimore: Williams & Wilkins, 1977, p. 320.
5. Chou TC. Electrocardiography in Practice. New York: Grune & Stratton, 1979, p. 468.
6. Beregovich J, et al. Management of acute myocardial infarction complicated by advanced atrioventricular block. Am J Cardiol. 1969;23:54.
7. Jackson AK, Bashour FA. Cardiac arrhythmias in acute myocardial infarction. I. Complete heart block and its natural history. Dis Chest. 1967;51:31.
8. Scherf D, Dix JH. The effects of posture on A-V conduction. Am Heart J. 1952;43:494.

FIG. 36.

A – Complete A-V block. Note plentiful P waves, regular ventricular rhythm at 24/min, and changing relationship between Ps and QRSs.

B – This sort of rhythm is often diagnosed as complete A-V block, but a better term is "block/acceleration dissociation." Certainly there is block, and certainly there is no conduction; but the ventricular rate (68/min) is too fast to afford optimal opportunity for conduction.

C – Complete A-V dissociation (bottom strip) produced by pacing a patient with only first degree block (top strip) slightly faster than his sinus rate. (Reproduced with permission from Langendorf R, Pick A. Am J Cardiol 1971;28:516.)

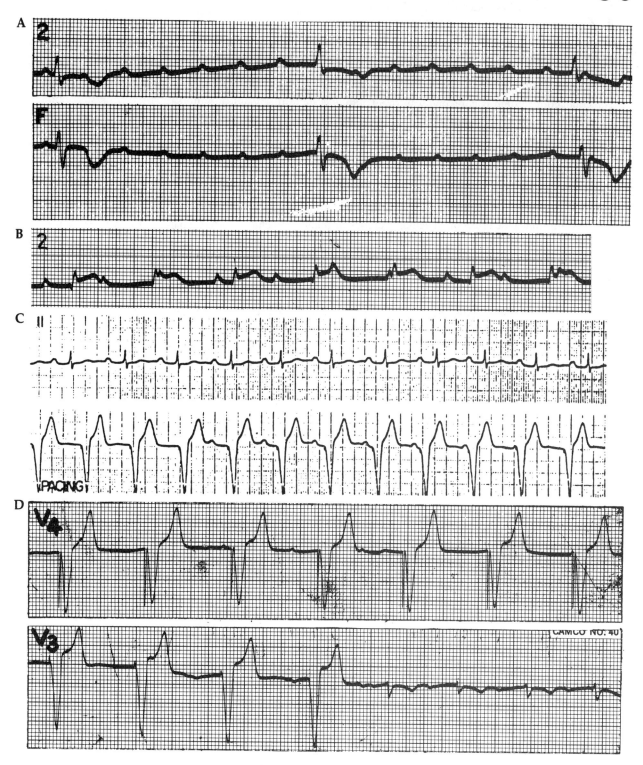

36

FIG. 36. (*continued*)

D – Top strip: Complete dissociation between sinus rhythm at 78/min and paced rhythm at 62/min. Clearly A-V block is present, no doubt aided and abetted by the effects of concealed retrograde conduction from the paced ventricular rhythm. **Bottom strip:** When a sinus impulse happens to arrive at the precisely critical moment (R-P interval), it captures the ventricles and reveals that the underlying block is only first degree. (Reproduced from Marriott HJ. Practical Electrocardiography. 8th ed. Baltimore: Williams & Wilkins, 1988).

37 RETROGRADE ANTICS

The conduction system is not a one-way street, although its traffic flow is usually anterograde. In fact, retrograde conduction of ectopic ventricular impulses is quite common. With use of an esophageal electrode, Kistin and Landowne demonstrated that 45% of ventricular extrasystoles sent their impulses all the way back to the atria (1). If that proportion of ectopic ventricular impulses succeed in reaching the atria, you can be sure that an additional fraction climbs as far as the A-V junction.

Figure 37-A illustrates a ventricular extrasystole with retrograde conduction to the atria. Figure 37-B illustrates the effect of an ectopic ventricular impulse reaching the A-V junction. Retrograde penetration of the junction leaves it refractory so that the P-R interval of the ensuing sinus beat is prolonged. Since the only visible evidence that the A-V junction has been invaded is the prolonged postectopic P-R interval, the retrograde conduction qualifies as "concealed" (see #45).

Figure 37-C illustrates the progressive effect of repeated concealed retrograde conduction during interpolated ventricular bigeminy simulating an A-V Wenckebach period.

Figures 37-D, E and F illustrate examples of retrograde conduction occurring during various ectopic ventricular rhythms—AIVR, paced rhythm and ventricular tachycardia.

In a significant minority of patients with complete A-V block, the impulse can go "uphill," but not "downhill." Figure 37-G is a short strip from a patient with complete A-V block showing several blocked atrial impulses, but the last ventricular impulse is conducted retrogradely to the atria (arrow). Such "atrial capture" is said to be present in 20% to 30% of complete anterograde A-V block (2,3).

REFERENCES

1. Kistin A, Landowne M. Retrograde conduction from ventricular premature contractions, a common occurrence in the human heart. Circulation. 1951;3:738.
2. Touboul P, et al. Retrograde conduction in complete atrioventricular block. Br Heart J. 1976;38:706.
3. Khalilullah M, et al. Unidirectional complete heart block. Am Heart J. 1979;97:608.

FIG. 37.

A – The third beat is a VPB with retrograde conduction to the atria.

B – The P-R interval of the sinus beat following the VPB is prolonged because of concealed retrograde conduction from the ventricular ectopic into the junction. This leaves the junction partially refractory so that the next descending impulse is delayed in transit.

C – Interpolated ventricular bigeminy with concealed retrograde conduction from each VPB progressively lengthening successive P-R intervals—so simulating an A-V Wenckebach period.

D – After two sinus beats, an accelerated idioventricular rhythm from the RV takes over by usurpation and retrograde conduction to the atria begins with the second ectopic beat (arrows).

E – Paced rhythm with retrograde conduction to the atria. The sharply pointed positive P waves are typical of retrograde conduction in V1.

F – Ventricular tachycardia with 3:2 retrograde Wenckebach periods alternating with 2:1 retrograde conduction to the atria (see laddergram).

G – Complete A-V block with retrograde "atrial capture." An inverted retrograde P wave is evident following the last ventricular beat (arrow).

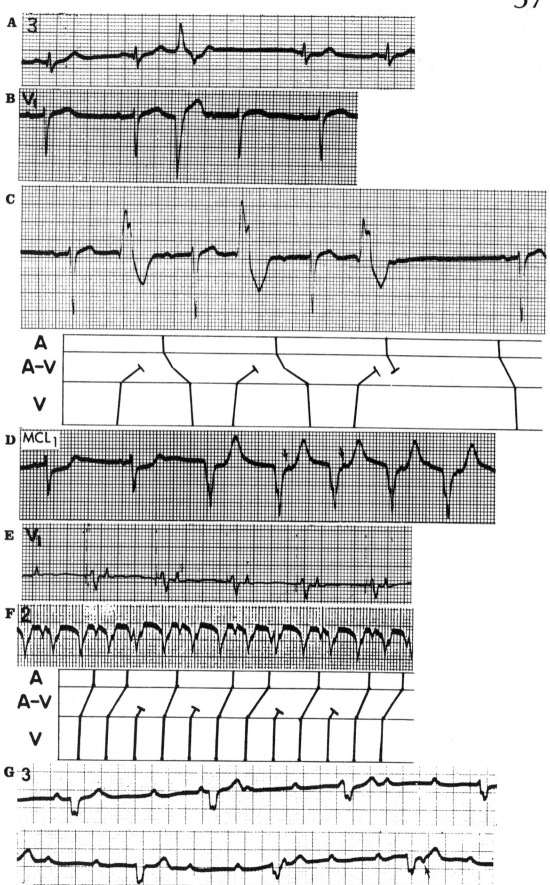

37

A 3

B V₁

C

A
A-V
V

D MCL₁

E V₁

F 2

A
A-V
V

G 3

38 DISSOCIATION VS. BLOCK

It is important not to confuse A-V dissociation with A-V block. A-V dissociation is exactly what it says: the independent beating of atria and ventricles—no more, no less (1). Block is one of the causes of A-V dissociation (Fig. 38-A), but it is not its synonym. There are three other causes of A-V dissociation that have nothing to do with block: (1) sinus bradycardia (Fig. 38-B), (2) acceleration of a subsidiary pacemaker (Fig. 38-C), and (3) pause-producers (Fig. 38-D). Of course A-V dissociation is often caused by a combination of two or more of the above four causes. Figure 38-E, for example, illustrates a combination of sinus bradycardia, junctional tachycardia and some degree of A-V block producing A-V dissociation.

REFERENCE

1. Pick A. A-V dissociation. A proposal for a comprehensive classification and consistent terminology. Am Heart J. 1963;66:147.

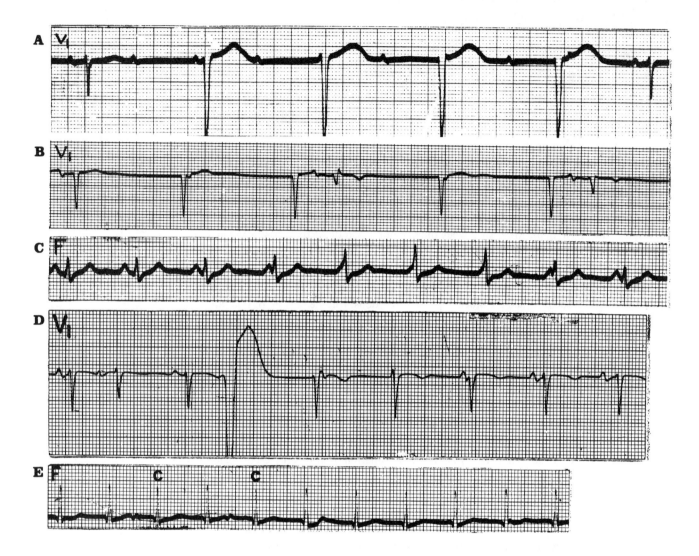

FIG. 38. THE FOUR CAUSES OF A-V DISSOCIATION.

A – A-V block: The second atrial impulse is blocked and this permits a subsidiary pacemaker, probably ventricular, to escape before the next atrial impulse can be conducted. A four-beat run of A-V dissociation results until, after the fourth ectopic beat, the R-P interval is long enough to allow A-V conduction to resume.

B – Sinus bradycardia: The sinus rhythm has a rate of 42/min that permits a junctional pacemaker to escape at the slightly faster rate of 45/min. After two escaped beats the ventricle is recaptured for one beat, with aberration of the captured beat. This sequence is again repeated.

C – Accelerated subsidiary pacemaker: After one conducted sinus beat, an accelerated junctional rhythm usurps control from the sinus and holds dissociated sway at a rate of 74/min to the end of the strip.

D – Pause-producer: After three beats—a sinus beat, an APB and an atrial escape beat—a VPB provides a long enough postectopic cycle for the junction to escape and dissociate for four beats at a rate of 70/min.

E – Sinus bradycardia (rate of 55/min) with some degree of A-V block and junctional tachycardia (rate of 102/min)—all due to digitalis. The third and fifth beats end slightly shorter cycles and are presumably conducted with prolonged P-R intervals; elsewhere, the two rhythms are dissociated.

39 CONCEALED CONDUCTION AGGRAVATING A-V BLOCK

We have seen in #37 how concealed retrograde conduction can simulate or enhance anterograde A-V block. Sometimes A-V block is made to look worse than it really is by the concealed conduction of antecedent anterograde ectopic atrial impulses. An example of this is seen in Fig. 39-A. In the top strip, the fact that the premature atrial impulse "b" is not conducted, even though the P' wave lands well beyond the T wave, suggests that significant A-V block is present. But the reason impulse "b" is not conducted is that impulse "a" has been conducted into the A-V junction leaving the junction refractory and thus preventing passage of impulse "b" (see laddergram). The fact that A-V conduction is not greatly impaired is attested to in the lower strip when the first of the pair of APBs is conducted, despite the fact that the P' wave is perched on top of the T wave. This prior conduction through the junction prevents acceptance of the second of the APB pair.

Again, in Figure 39-B, any number of the fluttering impulses are well beyond the T wave and yet are not conducted—and the block appears horrendous. But the reason for this failure of conduction late in the cycle is the concealed conduction of previous flutter impulses into the A-V junction leaving it refractory and so exaggerating the appearance of A-V blocks. Suspicion of the role played by antecedent flutter impulses is confirmed at the end of the strip where, at a sinus rate of 52/min, the A-V junction is capable of 1:1 conduction with only first degree A-V block.

Similarly, in the atrial fibrillation of Figure 39-C, the long cycle (which represents a ventricular rate of only 25/min) suggests that considerable A-V block is present. But the shortest cycles, before and after it—representing rates over 100/min—testify to competent A-V conduction. Obviously the long cycle is the result of superimposed repetitive concealed conduction of the fibrillatory impulses into the junction.

Thus it is important to realize that when you have apparent complete A-V block in the presence of atrial fibrillation (as in Fig. 39-D), the block may actually be comparatively mild and, if sinus rhythm is restored to the atria and concealed conduction thereby eliminated, such a heart may be entirely capable of conducting 1:1 at a reasonable sinus rate.

FIG. 39. ANTEROGRADE CONDUCTION IMPAIRED BY ANTECEDENT ANTEROGRADE CONCEALED CONDUCTION.

A – **Top strip.** Paired APBs: The second of each pair of APBs is not conducted because the first of each pair penetrates the A-V junction and leaves it refractory. This interpretation is confirmed in the **bottom strip** where the earlier APB is successfully conducted to the ventricles. In the top strip, the returning beats following the pairs of APBs are junctional escape beats.

B – At the end of the strip the conduction capability of 1:1 at a rate of 52/min with only first degree block is documented. Failure of conduction during the atrial flutter earlier in the strip is therefore attributable to the repetitive concealed conduction of atrial impulses into the A-V junction that always occurs with atrial flutter.

C – Similar situation during atrial fibrillation as in Figure 39-B. Judging by cycles earlier and later in the strip, conduction at a rate of 100/min is possible. The long cycle represents a rate of only 25/min and is the result of concealed conduction into the junction of fibrillatory impulses.

D – Atrial fibrillation with "complete" A-V block.

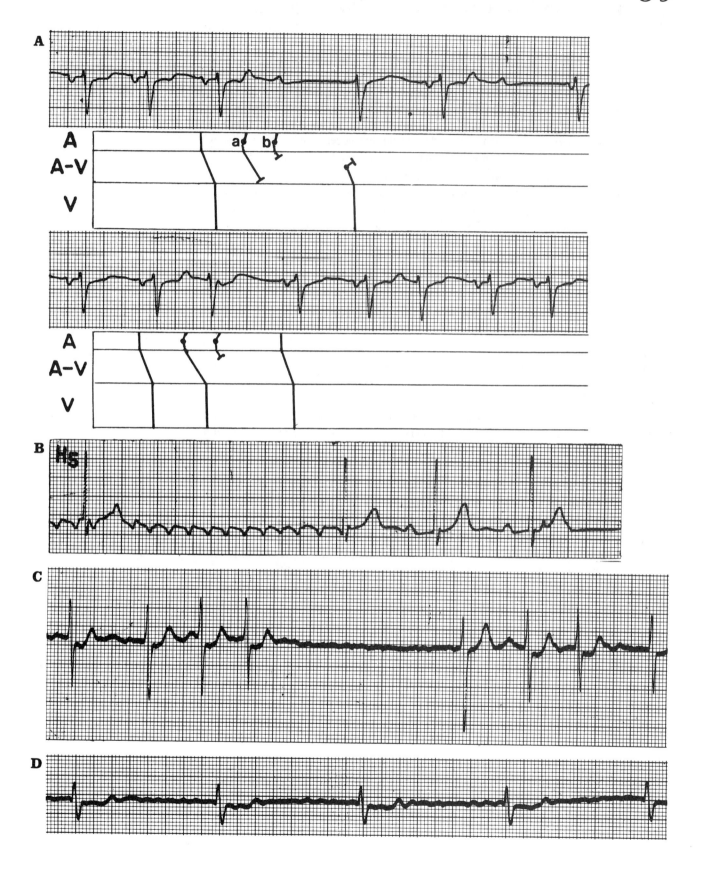

A

A
A-V
V

a b

A
A-V
V

B HS

C

D

CONCEALED CONDUCTION AGGRAVATING A-V BLOCK   95

40 CAPTURE(D) BEATS: TERMINOLOGY

Capture(d) beats, i.e., conducted beats interrupting A-V dissociation, are both fascinating and important. There are points to be made about their terminology, their recognition, and their value in diagnosis. When the atria and ventricles have been beating independently and then an atrial impulse is suddenly conducted, that conducted beat is a so-called captured beat. Because the ventricles are captured by the sinus impulse, the phenomenon is also referred to as ventricular capture. It is often erroneously, and quite illogically, called "sinus capture." Sinus, or atrial capture can indeed occur; but this is what happens when a retrograde impulse from an independently beating junctional or ventricular pacemaker suddenly controls the atria (see Fig. 37-G).

41 CAPTURE(D) BEATS: THEIR RECOGNITION

The way to recognize ventricular capture is not by finding an appropriate P-R interval, but rather by detecting a shortening of the R-R interval (ventricular cycle). This is perfectly logical because autonomous junctional or ventricular pacemakers usually beat with clockwork regularity. Therefore, any unexpected shortening of the ventricular cycle is strongly suggestive that the regularity of the independent rhythm has been interrupted by A-V conduction, and that an atrial impulse has managed to get through to the ventricles before the next independent beat is due. Four examples are shown in Figures 41-A to D.

Capture beats may be easily recognized because of their marked prematurity and readily observed preceding P waves at a conductible interval, as in Figures 41-A and 38-B. On other occasions, capture beats may be less obvious though still recognizable without precise measurement (Fig. 41-B); or they may be discernible only by careful measurement of the R-R intervals (Figs. 41-C and D).

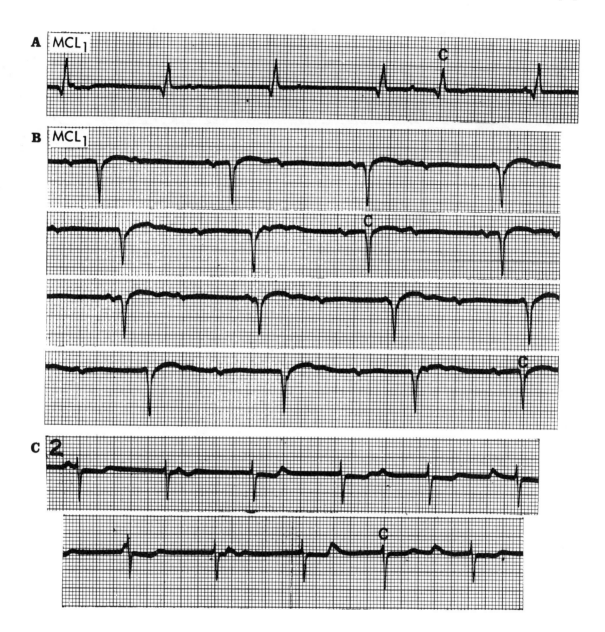

FIG. 41. CAPTURED BEATS

A – A-V dissociation due to sinus bradycardia in a patient with old anteroseptal infarction and RBBB. As a result of the sinus bradycardia (rate of 44/min), a junctional pacemaker escapes at a somewhat faster rate. The fifth beat (C) is a ventricular capture conducted with first degree A-V block.

B – In this patient with obvious A-V block and slow escape rhythm, the ventricular cycles in the top strip give the R-R interval of the junctional rhythm. Simple inspection, without precise measurement, identifies the third beat in the middle strip and the last beat in the bottom strip as ending somewhat shorter cycles. These beats are preceded by P waves at a conductible distance and are therefore ventricular captures. This illustrates that one cannot identify capture beats by P-R intervals alone because several other P-R intervals are certainly in the conductible range (e.g., first two P-R intervals in the top strip, last P-R interval in the second strip).

C – This tracing illustrates a capture beat that is almost impossible to recognize without meticulous measurement. The last beat in the top strip presents a plausible P-R interval; but careful measurement of the R-R interval reveals that the only capture beat is the fourth beat in the bottom strip (C).

41

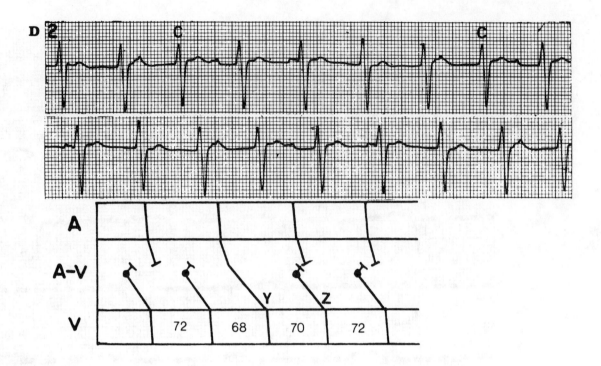

FIG. 41. (*continued*)

D – This tracing illustrates the impossibility of recognizing capture without precise measurement of R-R intervals. No unaided eye could recognize that every fifth beat ends a cycle shorter than the intervening ones. Surprisingly, the capture beats (the first two of which are labeled "C") turn out to be those that follow P waves perched on T waves.

This also illustrates the point that when two consecutive cycles are shorter than the dominant cycle, only the first can be regarded as definitely captured (see laddergram).

If the cycle of the independent pacemaker is consistently 72, then the sudden shortening to 68 is a sure sign of ventricular capture. But if the next cycle is also shorter than 72 (in this case 70), this is not firm evidence for another capture because the shortening of the "70" cycle may be due to delayed conduction of the beat that begins the cycle (Y)—as diagramed here—rather than to prematurity of the beat ending it (Z). This same point is again illustrated in Figure 42-D.

42 REWARD FOR CAPTURE

The diagnostic information contained in the lowly captured beat can be crucial. Tracings such as those in Figure 42 are often diagnosed as high-grade A-V block, of which inadequate definitions abound, and this over-diagnosis is one of the situations in which pacemakers have been overused. The importance of the captured beat is that it provides a better picture of the patient's conduction capability than all the nonconducted beats combined because a captured (conducted) beat immediately reveals what the patient needs for conduction. Let's examine that claim in some detail.

98   MOSTLY BLOCKS

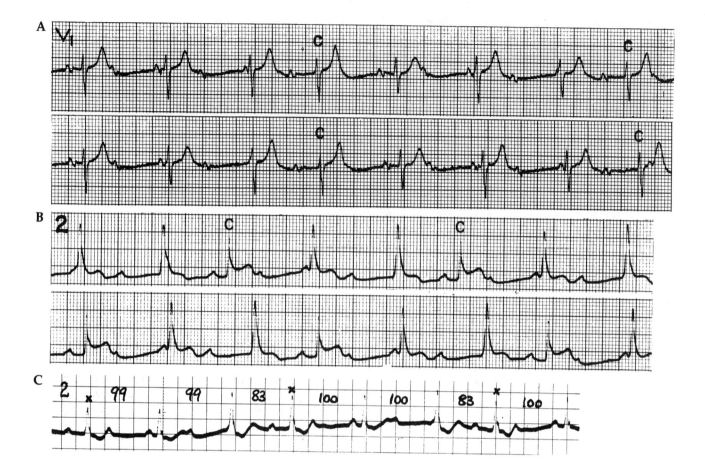

FIG. 42.

A – Block/acceleration dissociation with an atrial rate of 114/min and a junctional rate of 60/min, and with four ventricular captures (C). Note that the R-P/P-R ratio of the four captured beats is 48/32, 51/29, 50/30 and 45/41. Whenever the R-P interval is shorter than 45, no conduction occurs; nor does it occur after a longer R-P if the junctional beat preempts conduction. Following each conducted beat, the next R-P interval is short because of the accelerated atrial rate. To ensure conduction of every beat, every R-P interval would have to be at least 45, which would necessitate an atrial rate equal to the cycle of the captured beats, i.e., 70 to 75/min.

B – Block/acceleration dissociation with an atrial rate of 108/min, a junctional rate of 60/min, and five ventricular captures. The shortest cycles (77 to 79) are clearly the ones that end with ventricular capture. And because these cycles represent a rate of 75 to 76/min, that is the atrial rate at which one can predict 1:1 A-V conduction.

C – Block/acceleration dissociation with an atrial rate of 106/min, a ventricular rate of 60/min, and two ventricular captures (x). The shortest cycles (83) represent a rate of 74/min. Therefore, at this atrial rate, 1:1 conduction is possible.

42

In Figure 42-A, you see a tracing in which there is evident A-V block leading to A-V dissociation. In this sample of the tracing there are 28 P waves, but only four of the atrial impulses are conducted to the ventricles to produce captured beats (C). Thus, we have evident A-V block with only a small minority of the beats being conducted. This situation fulfills many published, but inadequate, definitions for high-grade or advanced A-V block, e.g., "a form of second degree block in which alternate, or two or more consecutive impulses fail to be conducted (1)." There is no mention of atrial rate, no consideration of why conduction failed. By this definition, all of the examples of block/acceleration in Figure 42 are high-grade, yet, as we will see, they all represent comparatively minor A-V block.

If the evidence afforded by the captured beats is taken advantage of, instead of concentrating on the fact that the vast majority of atrial impulses are not conducted, it is clear that the block is relatively mild—anything but high-grade. In fact, by looking at the cycles ending with captures and noting what rate these cycles represent, it takes only a few seconds to assess the situation. In this case the cycles represent a rate ranging from 70 to 75/min. One can now proclaim that if only the patient could have an atrial rate of 70 to 75/min, he would conduct every atrial impulse with a somewhat prolonged P-R interval and would then have mere "first degree" A-V block. In other words, the severity of the block is the equivalent of only first degree block at a rate of 70–75/min—mild block indeed!

To understand the reasoning, one must keep the following facts in mind: (1) the faster the atrial and/or ventricular rate, the greater the embarrassment to A-V conduction; (2) in all subjects with incomplete A-V block, there is always a critical R-P interval flagging the boundary between conduction and nonconduction, i.e., when the R-P interval is shorter than this critical length, conduction fails; whereas, when the R-P interval ranges beyond this boundary, conduction succeeds (unless, of course, the next independent beat obstructs its path).

With these facts in mind, let's examine the captured beats in Figure 42-A. The R-P/P-R measurements of the four capture beats are 48/32, 51/29, 50/30, 45/41 (Note the typical reciprocal relationship of type I block). Thus, for conduction to occur, this patient needs an R-P interval of at least 45, complemented by a somewhat prolonged P-R interval. Now consider what a handicap an accelerated atrial rate is to A-V conduction—because, following one of the conducted beats (C), the faster the atrial rate the shorter the next R-P interval, and therefore the less the likelihood of A-V conduction. Judging by the manifest requirements of the four captured beats, for consecutive conduction to occur, the R-P interval following the captured beat must again be at least 45; and this would necessitate an atrial rate of 75/min or less. Thus one can stipulate with confidence that, if the atrial rate were 75/min, every atrial impulse would be conductible because every R-P interval would be adequate. A simple, quick way of arriving at the required atrial rate is just to look at the rate represented by the cycle ending with a captured beat.

Now, without first reading the legends, apply these principles to figures 42-B to D and decide in each at what atrial rate 1:1 A-V conduction could be expected.

REFERENCE

1. WHO/ISC Task Force. Definition of terms related to cardiac rhythm. Am Heart J. 1978;95:796.

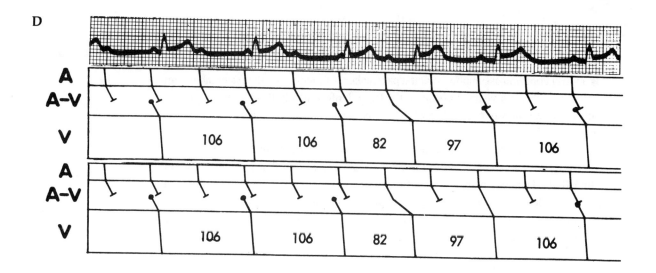

FIG. 42. (*continued*)

D – Block/acceleration dissociation with an atrial rate of 110/min, a ventricular rate of 57/min, and ventricular capture. The shortest cycle is 82, ending with the captured beat and representing a rate of 74/min. At this atrial rate, one can predict the capability of 1:1 A-V conduction. The next cycle is also shorter than the basic cycle (97 vs. 106), and may represent a second capture beat (lower laddergram). Conversely, its cycle may be foreshortened by the delayed conduction of the preceding captured beat (upper laddergram; also see Fig. 41-D).

43 PACEMAKER TREACHERY: NO BLIPS

It is a fairly common assumption that if a pacemaker is functioning, the pacemaker stimulus will always leave a visible imprint on the ECG. Unfortunately this is not true. Figure 43-A illustrates a runaway pacemaker whose "blips" are plain to see in lead aVF but quite invisible in lead 1.

Figure 43-B chronicles a near-disaster. The patient had received a temporary pacemaker on standby shortly after admission to the CCU with acute myocardial infarction complicated by LBBB. The demand pacemaker did a double disservice by operating in the fixed-rate (VOO) mode and by not producing the expected blips in the monitoring lead. Consequently, the paced beats were mistaken for ventricular extrasystoles and were treated in vain (and in vein) with increasingly toxic doses of lidocaine and procainamide. The source of the ectopic beats was recognized only when someone noted that the ectopic beats showed the features of parasystole (bottom strip)—varied coupling with constant interectopic intervals (see #6). Knowing that a fixed-rate pacemaker behaves exactly like parasystole, the attendants deduced that the pacemaker's demand mode was faulty and that its stimulus artifacts were invisible in the monitoring lead.

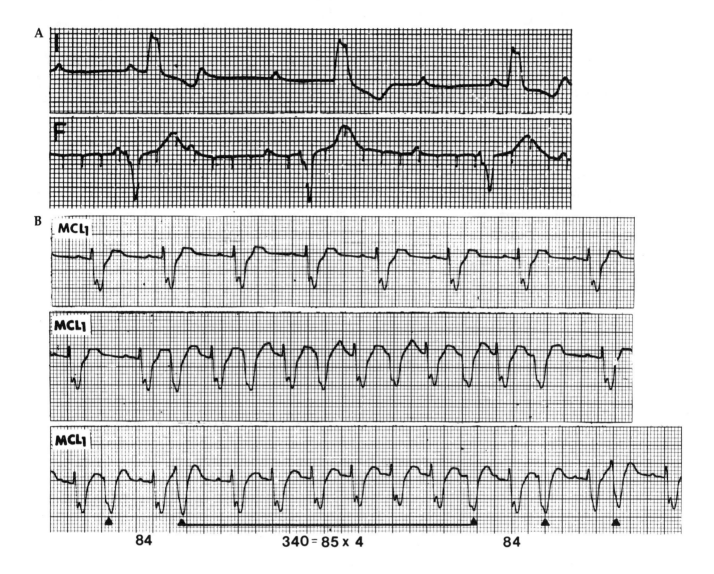

43

FIG. 43.

A – Complete A-V block with idioventricular escape rhythm at a rate of 36/min, complicated by runaway pacemaker whose stimulus artifacts are clearly visible in lead aVF but invisible in lead 1.

B – **Top strip:** sinus tachycardia (145/min) with 2:1 A-V block and LBBB. **Middle strip:** sinus tachycardia with 2:1 A-V block and LBBB complicated by a run of interpolated right ventricular bigeminy. **Bottom strip:** The coupling interval of ventricular ectopic beats (arrows) varies while the interectopic intervals remain constant at 84–85 (parasystolic behavior suggesting the operation of a fixed rate pacemaker). Sinus tachycardia has slowed somewhat—now 130/min—with 1:1 A-V conduction in the middle of the strip and the interval between ectopic beats (340) a multiple of the pacemaker's cycle (84–85).

44 PACEMAKER TREACHERY: FAULTY SENSING?

In patients with RBBB wearing a permanent demand pacemaker, the stimulus artifact often lands in the middle of the QRS complex, which may be interpreted as faulty sensing. But remember that if RBBB is present and the electrode is in the right ventricle, the only way the inhibiting impulse can reach the electrode is down the left bundle branch and through the septum. It may take 8 or 9 hundredths of a second after the beginning of the QRS before the electrode is reached, and therefore a pacemaker blip landing in the first half or two-thirds of a QRS manifesting RBBB may not imply abnormal sensing.

For comparison, a genuine example of faulty sensing is reproduced in Figure 44B.

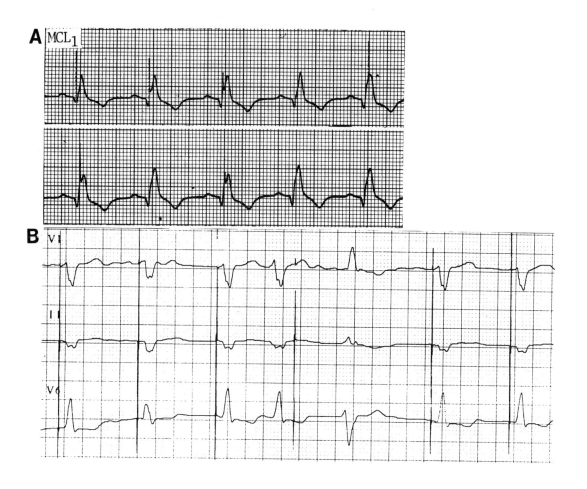

44

FIG. 44. FAULTY SENSING: SUPPOSED AND GENUINE

A – RV demand pacemaker in presence of RBBB: normal. (Reproduced from Marriott HJ. Practical Electrocardiography. 8th ed. Baltimore: Williams & Wilkins, 1988. p. 413.)

B – Against a background of atrial fibrillation, after three successfully paced beats, an early, nonpaced beat appears which, instead of being recognized (sensed) by the pacemaker, is overlooked. The next pacemaker stimulus therefore lands on the ST segment at the end of its established automatic interval. This failure to sense is followed by another natural beat which is appropriately sensed. The pacemaker is inhibited and waits for another full automatic interval before firing again.

45 A TALE OF TWO CYCLES

A useful principle in arrhythmic diagnosis is as follows: When there are two families of cycles, one shorter and one longer, you should assume—till proved otherwise—that the shorter cycle is the basic cycle and that something has lengthened the longer one. As a result of this principle, the way to approach such a tracing is to measure the shorter cycle and subtract it from the longer cycle backwards; i.e., begin at the end of the longer cycle and, measuring backwards the interval of the shorter cycle to see if a recognizable lengthening influence is encountered—"the grand thing is to be able to reason backwards!"(1)

In Figure 45-A, there are two families of paced cycles: the shorter measure 0.98 s and the longer 1.38 s. The changing cycle lengths suggest pacemaker malfunction. But if you measure 0.98 s back from the end of one of the longer cycles, you engage the T wave, which clearly means that the oversensitive pacemaker was sensing T waves. Figure 45-B illustrates the same phenomenon in a child. The 6th and 7th paced cycles are measurably longer than the rest (0.94 s vs. 0.64 s). If you measure backwards 0.64 s from the end of the 6th and 7th cycle, you land precisely on the preceding T waves.

And the same principle applies in natural rhythms that have two families of cycles. In Figure 45-C, the shorter cycles measure 1.17 to 1.27 s, and the longer cycles are about 1.53 s. The shortest cycles of all result from ventricular captures thanks to supernormal conduction. In the bottom strip, if the shorter cycle (1.27 s) is measured backwards from the end of the longer cycle, it becomes evident that the cycle has been lengthened by (concealed) supernormal conduction of the atrial impulse (arrow) into the junction.

Definition: Supernormal conduction is conduction that is better than expected, better earlier in the ventricular cycle than later (it is not better than normal, as the term implies).

REFERENCE

1. Sherlock Holmes in The Sign of Four.

FIG. 45.

A – Right ventricular demand pacemaker intermittently sensing the T wave.

B – Demand pacemaker sensing the T wave in two consecutive cycles in a 4-year-old child with congenital complete A-V block.

C – A-V block with junctional escape rhythm at a rate of 48/min and interrupted once in each strip with supernormal A-V conduction. **Top strip:** The fourth beat manifests supernormal A-V conduction of the sinus impulse (P wave on T) with unchanged intraventricular conduction. **Middle strip:** The fourth beat again manifests supernormal A-V conduction (P wave on ST) but with RBBB aberration. **Bottom strip:** After the third beat, the next sinus impulse (arrow) is conducted into the junction, discharging the junctional pacemaker and postponing its next beat (see laddergram). This is an example of *concealed* supernormal conduction.

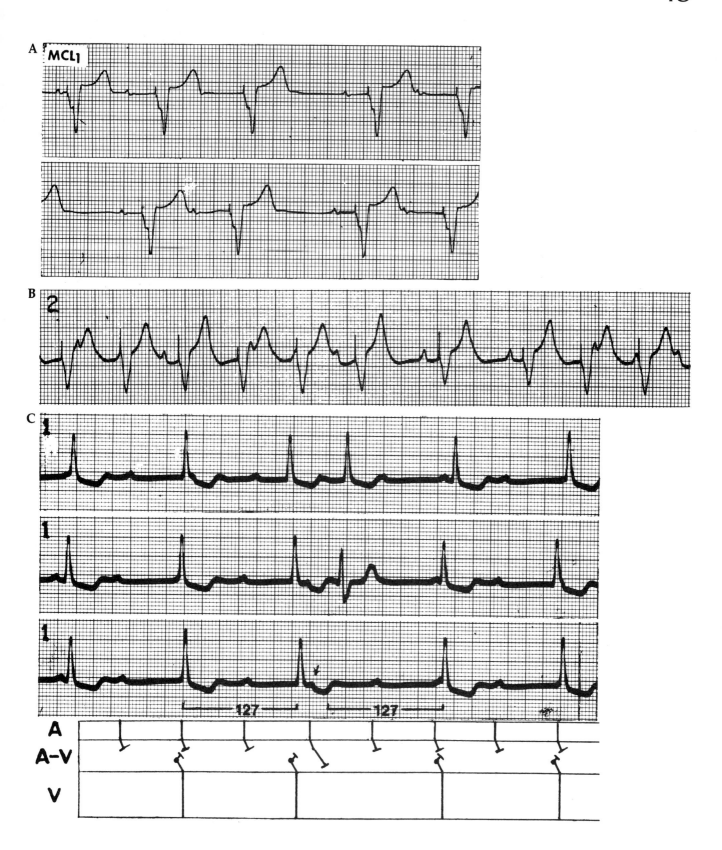

45

PART 4
12-LEAD REVELATIONS

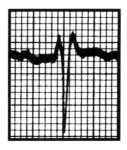

46 MITRAL STENOSIS: THE LEAD 1 CLUE

The likely tip-off to mitral stenosis in the 12-lead tracing is the combination of left atrial with right ventricular enlargement (Fig. 46-A) because this is otherwise an unlikely combination.

A subtle expression of this clue may be found in standard lead 1: a P wave whose height rivals that of the accompanying R wave (Fig. 46-B).

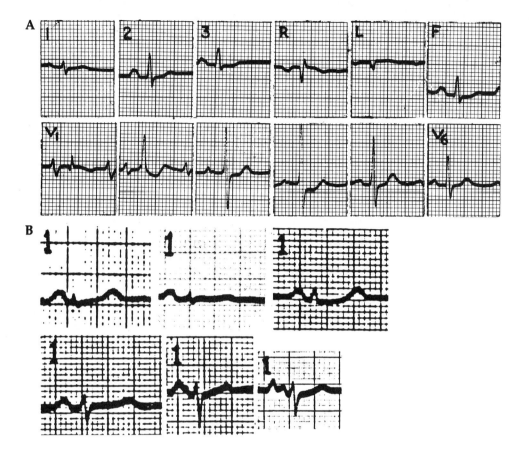

46

FIG. 46.

A – 12-lead tracing from a white woman with severe mitral stenosis showing evidence of left atrial (huge negative P-terminal force in V1) with RVH (dominant R in V1 and V2).

B – Lead 1 from six patients with mitral stenosis showing prominent P wave rivaling or exceeding the height of the R wave.

47 MITRAL STENOSIS: THE AXIS/FIBRILLATION CLUE

Another pair of findings suggestive of mitral stenosis is the combination of atrial fibrillation with right axis deviation (Fig. 47-A-C). Persistently increased left atrial pressure, resulting in left atrial enlargement, is the trigger that initiates atrial fibrillation, while the right axis deviation is part and parcel of the pattern of RVH.

Of course this combination may be seen in other situations; for example, in an elderly hypertensive patient with cor pulmonale, or in an adult with atrial septal defect. But in the first four or five decades of life, and particularly in females, the overwhelming diagnostic probability is mitral stenosis.

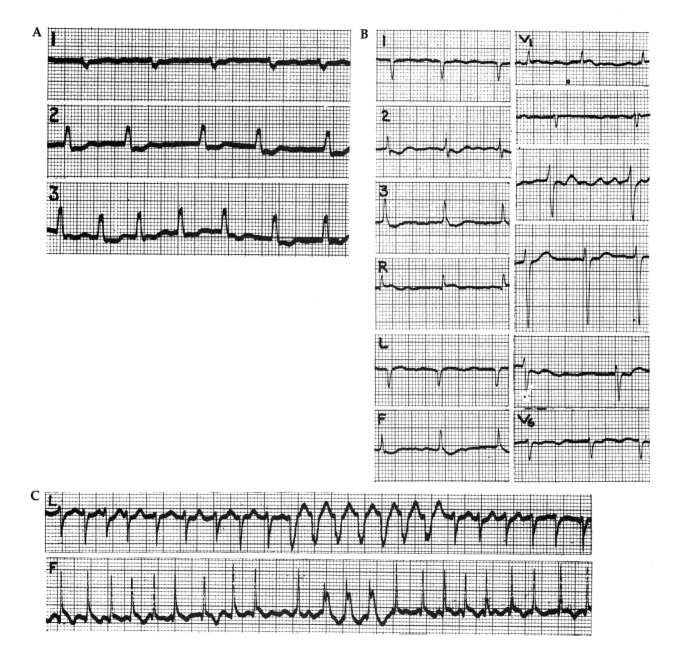

47

FIG. 47. ATRIAL FIBRILLATION AND RIGHT AXIS DEVIATION IN THREE PATIENTS WITH MITRAL STENOSIS.

A – Atrial fibrillation and right axis deviation.

B – Note the evidence of RVH in the V leads.

C – The rapid ventricular response (200/min) is complicated by runs of ventricular aberration in the middle of each strip.

48 AXIS DEVIATION IN LBBB

LBBB is almost always associated with either a normal QRS axis or left axis deviation. The presence of marked left axis deviation usually implies additional disease besides the sick bundle branch and worsens the prognosis (1,2). At times it may mean that the LBBB is incomplete and is associated with complete block in the anterior fascicle (left anterior hemiblock) (3).

When LBBB is accompanied by right axis deviation (Fig. 48-A), the combination is highly suggestive of a dilated or congestive cardiomyopathy (4).

REFERENCES

1. Dhingra RC, et al. Significance of left axis deviation in patients with chronic left bundle-branch block. Am J Cardiol. 1978;2:551.
2. Swiryn S, et al. Electrocardiographic determinants of axis during left bundle branch block; study in patients with intermittent left bundle branch block. Am J Cardiol. 1980;6:53.
3. Rosenbaum MB. The hemiblocks, Tampa Tracings, 1970, p. 162.
4. Nikolic G, Marriott HJ.Left bundle branch block with right axis deviation: a marker of congestive cardiomyopathy. J Electrocardiol. 1985;18:395.

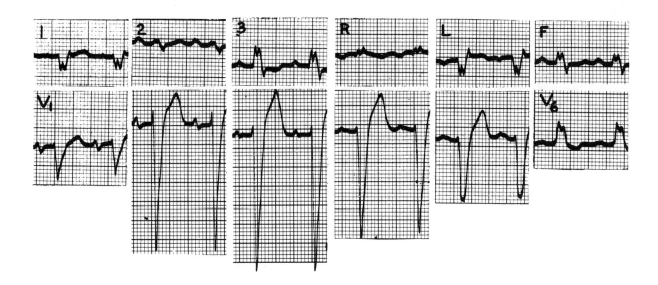

48

FIG. 48. LBBB WITH RIGHT AXIS DEVIATION FROM A 44-YEAR-OLD BLACK MAN WITH COR BOVINUM BECAUSE OF A DILATED PRIMARY CARDIOMYOPATHY.

49 LBBB WITH Q WAVES

It is well known that, in the presence of LBBB, the initial q in left lateral leads (1, aVL, V5–6) of septal activation disappears. The reason for this is that if LBBB develops, the septum can no longer be initially activated from the left side, as it normally is. If, therefore, q waves are found in these leads, it is virtually specific for myocardial infarction. Interestingly, as they demonstrated at the Mayo Clinic decades ago that, although the q waves are in lateral leads, the infarction is invariably anteroseptal (1).

Although the presence of such q waves should make one suspicious of an associated myocardial infarction, subsequent autopsy studies (2,3) have demonstrated that q waves may be found in the absence of any post mortem evidence of an infarct.

REFERENCES

1. Rhoades DV, et al. The electrocardiogram in the presence of myocardial infarction and intraventricular block of the left bundle-branch block type. Am Heart J. 1961;62:735.
2. Scott RC. Left bundle branch block—a clinical assessment. Am Heart J. 1965;70:691.
3. Horan LG, et al. The significance of diagnostic Q waves in the presence of bundle branch block. Chest. 1970;58:214.

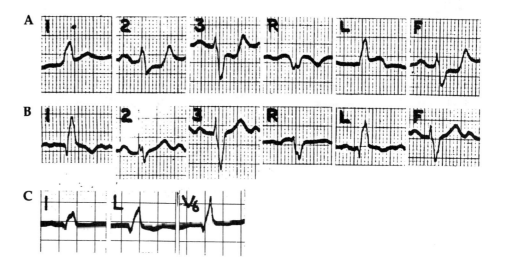

49

FIG. 49. TWO EXAMPLES OF LBBB WITH ABNORMAL Q WAVES IN LATERAL LEADS.

A – ST elevation in 1 and aVL with reciprocal depression in 2, 3 and aVF make the diagnosis of acute anterior infarction despite the presence of LBBB.

B – One day later, diagnostic Q waves have developed in 1 and aVL.

C – Another patient showing Q waves diagnostic of anterior infarction in leads 1, aVL, and V6, in the presence of LBBB.

50 LBBB AND MYOCARDIAL INFARCTION

It is often taught that myocardial infarction cannot be diagnosed in the presence of LBBB. This false doctrine appears to be based on the fact that the QRS changes of myocardial infarction seldom assert themselves in the presence of LBBB. This is because when LBBB and infarction are contemporaneous, there is a "tug-of-war" on the stylus. The infarction tries to produce Q waves but the LBBB doesn't want them; sometimes the infarction wins—as seen in #49—but usually it doesn't.

If, however, one concentrates on the repolarization moiety of the ventricular complex, it is a different story and diagnostic changes are observed in at least two-thirds of patients. Figures 50-A to D illustrate ST-T changes of acute myocardial injury superimposed upon LBBB.

REFERENCE

1. Sgarbossa EB, et al: Electrocardiographic diagnosis of evolving acute myocardial infarction in the presence of left bundle-branch block. N Engl J Med. 1996:334:482.

FIG. 50. FOUR EXAMPLES OF DIAGNOSABLE ACUTE MYOCARDIAL INFARCTION IN THE PRESENCE OF LBBB.

A – Monumental ST elevation in mid-precordial leads which could not be due to anything but acute injury. Note the more moderate elevation in leads 1, aVL and V5 where STs should be depressed in LBBB. Also note the tiny Q waves in leads 1 and aVL.

B – In addition to the convex-upward elevation of the ST segments in V leads, there are vicious Q waves in leads 1, aVL, V5 and V6.

C – The upward convexity of the elevated ST segments, combined with the tiny Q waves in leads 1 and aVL, are diagnostic of myocardial infarction.

D – Acute inferior wall myocardial infarction is documented by the ST elevation in leads 2, 3 and aVF (where, with upright QRSs in LBBB, they should be depressed), together with reciprocal ST depression in V2 and V3. Note that there are no diagnostic Q waves.

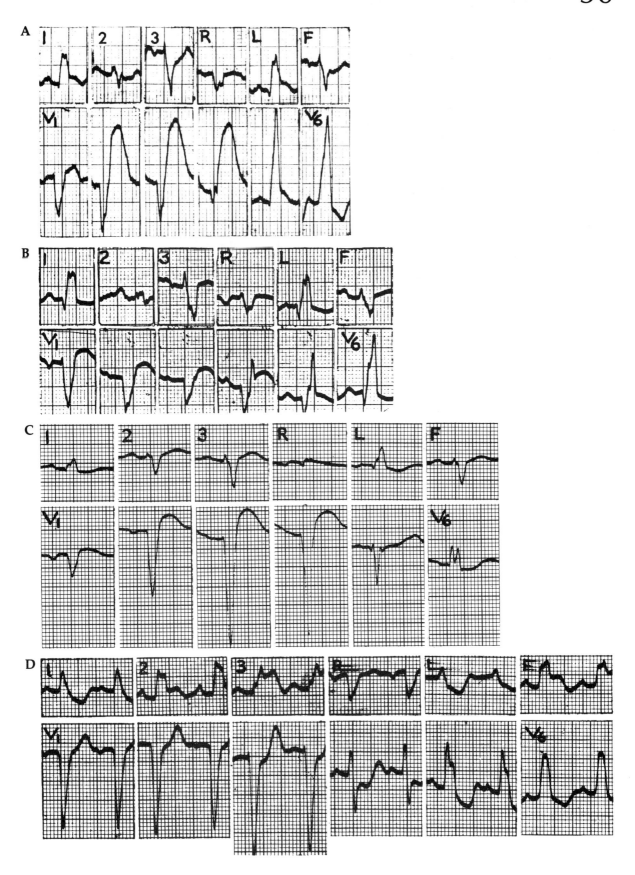

50

51 FIRST SIGN OF RBBB

Evidence of developing RBBB can be recognized in V1 before an R′ wave appears. The early signs are a shrinking S wave and a slurred upstroke of the S wave. In Figures 51-A and C there are two APBs, the first conducted with minor aberration, the second with RBBB aberration. Note that the main change in the first APB is a shrinkage of the S wave. In Figure 51-E, three junctional premature beats are depicted: the first two show two stages of S-shrinkage with full-blown RBBB in the third. Figure 51-B illustrates the progressive development of RBBB in successive sinus beats. Note that in the second beat, as the QS complex shrinks, notching develops in the upstroke. In Figure 51-D, the second APB shows RBBB, whereas the first illustrates both S-wave shrinkage and a notched upstroke. Finally, in Figure 51-F, as RBBB develops, the notch on the upstroke of the S wave rises higher and higher (first seven beats) until in the last two beats the notch pushes above the baseline and creates an r′.

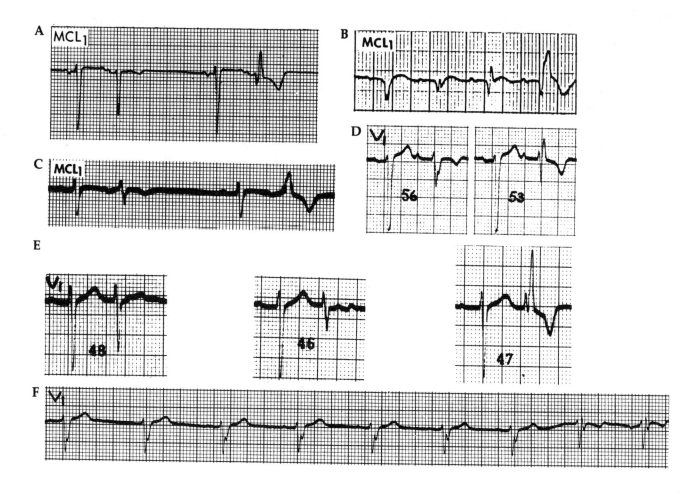

51

FIG. 51. SIX EXAMPLES (A TO F) ILLUSTRATING VARYING DEGREES OF RBBB (FOR DETAILED DESCRIPTION, SEE TEXT).

52 RATE-DEPENDENT Q WAVES

We have seen that the Q wave of infarction may show up better in ectopic ventricular beats than in conducted sinus beats (#2). Less well known is the fact that anteroseptal infarction Q waves may appear only in the presence of the faster rate at which rate-dependent RBBB develops. Rosenbaum published a classical example of this phenomenon (Fig. 52-A)(1).

REFERENCE

1. Rosenbaum MB, et al. Abnormal Q waves in right sided chest leads provoked by onset of right bundle-branch block in patients with anteroseptal infarction. Br Heart J. 1982;47:227.

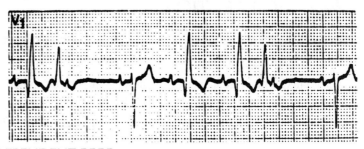

52

FIG. 52. RATE-DEPENDENT RBBB

A – The third and last beat, ending the longest cycles, are normally conducted. The fourth and fifth beat, ending shorter cycles, evoke RBBB and alone manifest the Q waves of anteroseptal infarction. (Reproduced with permission of author and publisher from Rosenbaum MB, Br Heart J 1982;47:227).

53 EARLY DIAGNOSIS OF INFERIOR INFARCTION

Acute inferior myocardial infarction can sometimes be diagnosed earliest by reciprocal changes. The likely-to-be-overlooked aVL lead can be especially helpful in the diagnosis.

Figure 53-A is from a 41-year-old woman who developed epigastric discomfort and visited an emergency department. The ECG changes were accepted by a cardiologist as "nonspecific ST-T abnormalities," the diagnosis of indigestion was made and she was sent home with an antacid. At 1:00 a.m. she had cardiac arrest, was brought to the emergency department, and was defibrillated. Unfortunately, the conversion was too late to save her brain and she was a cerebral vegetable. Two years later she was still alive but unable to look after her family of four children. The family brought suit and was rewarded with a sizable settlement. All of this could have been avoided if the changes in aVL (and other leads, see legend) had been recognized as highly suspicious of acute inferior infarction.

Three more acute inferior infarctions, with minimal if any indicative changes, but flagrant reciprocal changes, are shown in Figures 53 B to F. Note that in each case, the ST-T negativity in aVL is out of proportion to the size of the QRS.

FIG. 53. EARLY INFERIOR WALL MYOCARDIAL INFARCTION

A – The slight elevation of the ST segments in leads 2, 3, and aVF might well pass for normal; but the ST displacement in aVL, the horizontal ST segments in leads 1, V3, and V4, and the sharp-angled ST-T junctions in leads V2 to V4 are unequivocal abnormalities and represent "reciprocal" changes.

B – The ST elevation in leads 2, 3, and aVF are, again, equivocal, but the ST-T changes in aVL and the V leads are conclusively reciprocal.

C – This tracing, from the same patient 1 day later, confirms an evolving inferoposterior infarction.

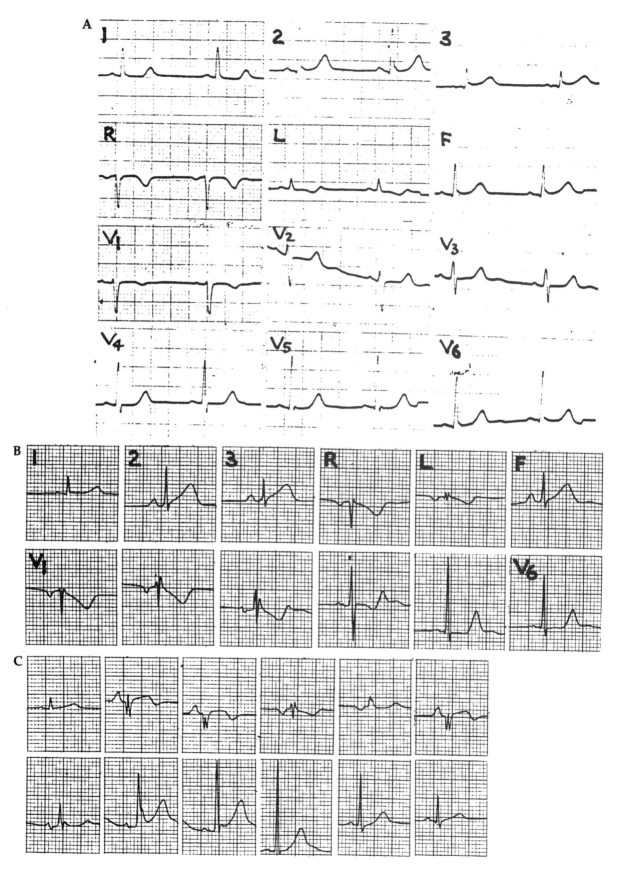

53

FIG. 53. *(continued)*

D – There is loss of the normal upward ST concavity in lead 3 and a hint of it in aVF, but no such loss in lead 2. Meanwhile, there is significant ST-T negativity in aVL, and V1–3 show reciprocal ST-T changes.

E – There is no sign of abnormality in the inferior leads, but leads 1 and aVL present typical reciprocal changes; while V2, V3 and V6 show ST horizontality and/or sharp-angled ST-T junctions.

F – Two days after the ECG in Figure 53-E was taken, evolutionary changes of inferior infarction are evident in leads 2 and 3.

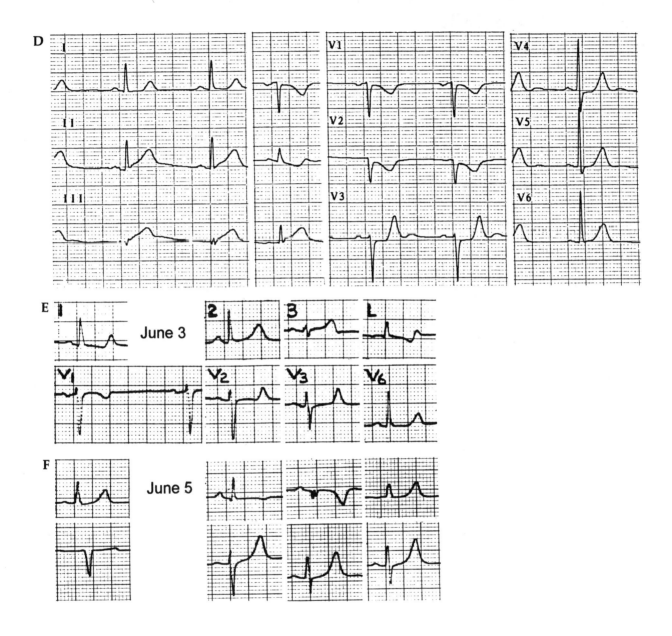

D

I   V1   V4
II   V2   V5
III V3   V6

E   1   June 3   2   3   L

V1   V2   V3   V6

F   June 5

54 INFERIOR INFARCTION AND ANTERIOR HEMIBLOCK

The diagnosis of concomitant inferior infarction with left anterior hemiblock (LAHB) has always been problematic because they can both produce significant left axis deviation. If the left axis deviation is caused by prominent Q waves, you know there has been an infarction but you are not sure if there is an associated LAHB. On the other hand, if the left axis shift is mediated by deep S waves, you know that you're dealing with anterior hemiblock but you cannot exclude a myocardial infarction.

Warner has proposed a neat device for recognizing LAHB complicating inferior infarction (1,2). Because, with LAHB, the vector loop terminally rotates counterclockwise (Fig. 54, top), it follows that the QRS must reach maximal positivity in lead aVL before it reaches its terminal peak in aVR. Therefore, if you record aVL and aVR simultaneously (preferably at accelerated paper speed), it will be easy to see whether or not the R wave in aVL reaches its peak before the R′ in aVR (Fig. 54, bottom). If it does, you know you are dealing with a complicating LAHB.

This ingenious device, however, despite the logic of it, requires independent confirmation before it can be accepted (3).

REFERENCES

1. Warner RA, et al. Improved electrocardiographic criteria for the diagnosis of left anterior hemiblock. Am J Cardiol. 1983;51:723.
2. Warner RA, et al. Electrocardiographic criteria for the diagnosis of combined inferior myocardial infarction and left anterior hemiblock. Am J Cardiol. 1983;51:718.
3. Antoniak T, et al. Value of Warner criteria for the diagnosis of left anterior hemiblock. Am J Noninvas Cardiol. 1989;3:48.

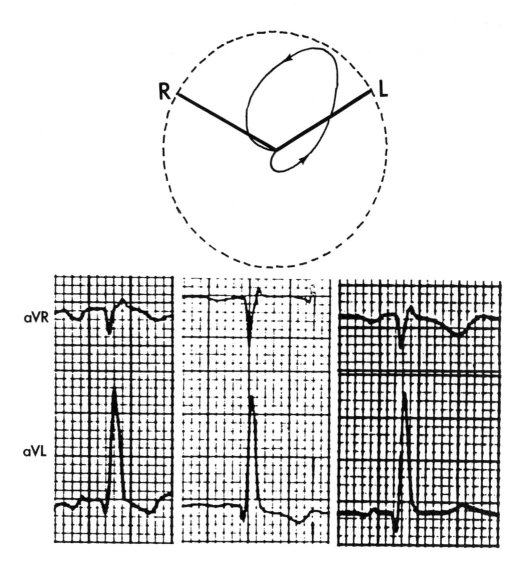

54

FIG. 54.

Top: Representation of the counterclockwise loop of left anterior hemiblock. Note that the vector scans the positive field of aVL before that of aVR and therefore the positive peak of aVL is reached before the positive peak of aVR.

Bottom: Leads aVR and aVL simultaneously recorded from three patients with left anterior hemiblock. The peak of the R wave in aVL in each case precedes that in aVR by 0.03 to 0.04 s.

55 RV INFARCTION

Although V4R is the most diagnostic single lead for recognizing the ST elevation of RV infarction (Fig. 55-A), a virtually diagnostic clue in the routine 12-lead tracing is the combination of elevated ST segments in lead V1 with reciprocal depression in V2 (Fig. 55-B and C)(1).

In fact, if you monitor with lead V1 or MCL1, you may get an early clue to RV infarction on the oscilloscope. If a patient has a known inferior wall myocardial infarction, even though the ST segment is clearly elevated in the monitoring lead (when you would expect it to be depressed in V1 as in Figure 55-D), there is a strong presumption that the right ventricle is also involved.

REFERENCE

1. Macfarlane PW, Lawrie TD. Comprehensive electrocardiology. Pergamon Press, NY 1989, p. 605.

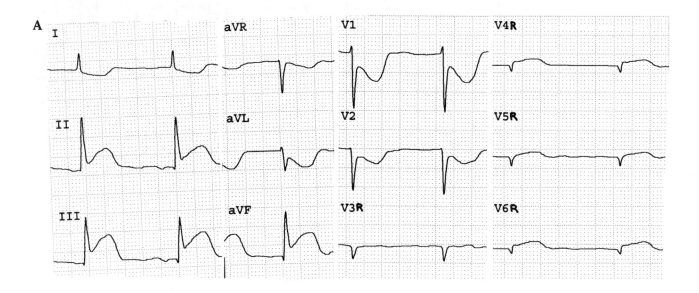

FIG. 55. FOUR EXAMPLES OF ACUTE INFERIOR MYOCARDIAL INFARCTION

In **A,** a right-sided series of precordial leads shows ST elevation in V4R through V6R, diagnostic of RV infarction. (Tracing courtesy Dr. William Nelson.) In **B** and **C,** the diagnosis can be made from the conventional 12-lead tracings thanks to the combination of ST elevation in V1 with reciprocal depression in V2. The rhythm in C is junctional bradycardia. In **D,** the ST is depressed in both V1 and V2 so that RV infarction cannot be recognized unless a series of right-sided leads reveals it (as in A above). (C and D are reproduced from Marriott HJ, Practical Electrocardiography. 8th ed. Baltimore, Williams & Wilkins, 1988.)

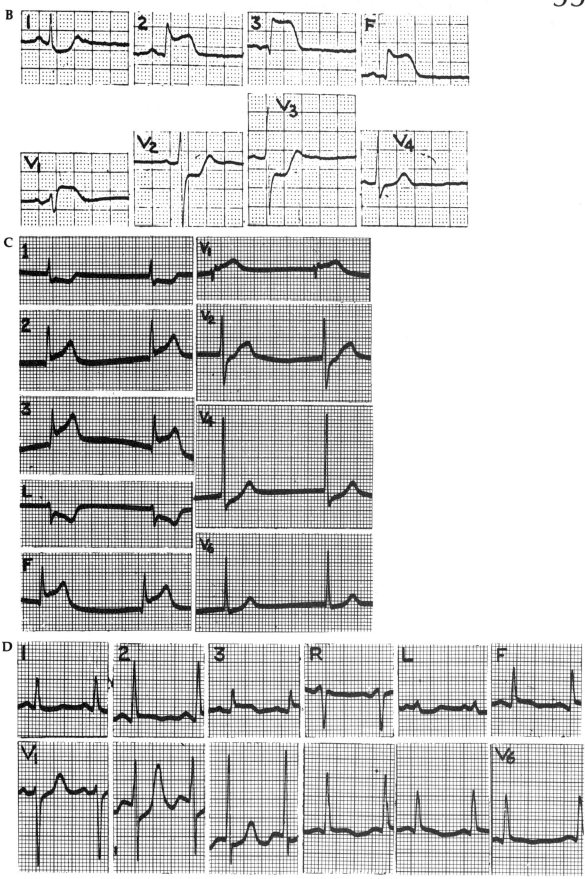

55

56 ESTIMATING RV PRESSURE FROM V1

In RV hypertrophy, the RV pressure can be estimated with reasonable accuracy from the QRS configuration in lead V1 (Table 56.1). If the pattern is qR, there is a 75% probability that the RV pressure exceeds LV pressure. If the pattern is rR, there is a 75% probability that RV and LV pressures are approximately equal. If the pattern is Rs, there is a 75% likelihood that the RV pressure is less than LV pressure.

TABLE 56.1.
RELATIONSHIP OF QRS PATTERN IN V_1 TO BALANCE OF PRESSURES
IN THE TWO VENTRICLES

V_1	RVP > LVP (22 CASES)	RVP = LVP (114 CASES)	RVP < LVP (85 CASES)
	78%	5%	—
	22%	77%	10%
	—	14%	75%
	—	4%	15%

57 CONGENITAL RIGHT VENTRICULAR HYPERTROPHY

Attention to QRS-T detail may help to distinguish between the RVH of pure pulmonic stenosis (PPS) and that of tetralogy of Fallot. In PPS, the R wave tends to remain dominant and the T wave inverted from V1 through V3 or V4 (Fig. 57-A). In a tetralogy on the other hand, the R wave tends to lose its dominance and the T wave tends to become upright, if not by V2 at least by V3 (Fig. 57-B).

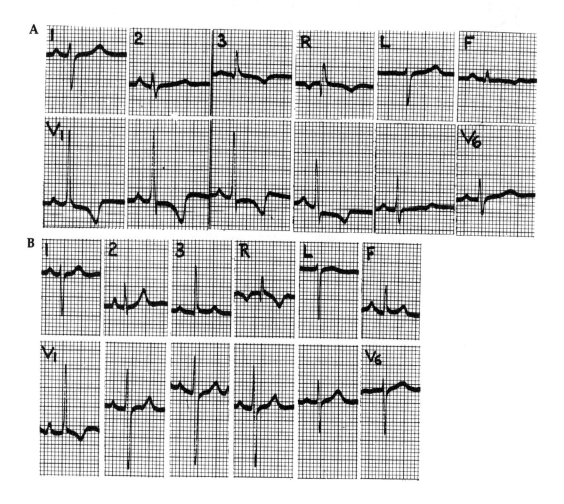

FIG. 57. CONGENITAL HEART DISEASE WITH RVH

A is from a 35-year-old woman with pure pulmonic stenosis (PPS) and RV pressure of 140 mm, whereas **B** is from a child with tetralogy of Fallot (TET). Note that in PPS, the R wave is dominant and T wave inverted from V1 to V4, whereas in the TET the T wave is upright and the S wave dominant in V2 to V4.

58 ACUTE COR PULMONALE

Many clues have been suggested for the diagnosis of pulmonary embolism. These include the classical McGinn-White S1-Q3 pattern, dominant S waves in all V leads, RBBB, and ST elevation in lead 3 with depression in leads 1 and 2 with "staircase" ascent in lead 2.

But a very simple and eye-catching clue is the presence of changes that suggest ischemic disease in inferior and anteroseptal leads simultaneously (Figs. 58-A and B, bottom panels). To put it aphoristically: *if you find yourself thinking of inferior ischemia, injury, or infarction as you scan the limb leads, but then in the precordial leads you favor anteroseptal ischemia, injury, or infarction, let it switch on a little cerebral light and suggest acute cor pulmonale.* The minimal change that should indicate the possibility is the abnormal inversion of the T wave in lead 3 and in V1 (Fig. 58-C, bottom panel). In both these leads, of course, the T wave can be normally inverted, so it requires inversion of abnormal depth to raise the suspicion. Anything that produces acute cor pulmonale—such as an overwhelming pneumonia (Fig. 58-E)—can produce a similar ECG. On rare occasions a comparable pattern may be found in chronic pulmonary artery obstruction (Fig. 58-D).

It is true that Levine has drawn attention to a similar pattern occurring in 6 out of 53 (12%) autopsied subendocardial infarctions (1); and the combination of inverted T waves in anteroseptal leads and in lead 3 and/or aVF may also be found in right ventricular arrhythmogenic dysplasia (2). Nevertheless, the inferior/anteroseptal conspiracy is otherwise uncommon and should always first evoke the suspicion of acute cor pulmonale.

REFERENCES

1. Levine HD. Subendocardial infarction in retrospect: pathologic, cardiographic, and ancillary features. Circulation. 1985;72:79.
2. Lemery R, et al. Nonischemic sustained ventricular tachycardia: clinical outcome in 12 patients with arrhythmogenic right ventricular dysplasia. J Am Coll Cardiol. 1989;14:96.

FIG. 58.

A – From a 50-year-old man with acute cor pulmonale. **Top panel:** Control normal tracing. **Bottom panel:** Two years later at the time of pulmonary embolism. Note the abnormal T-wave inversion in leads 3, aVF, and V1 to V3, associated with the sudden appearance of S waves everywhere.

B – From a 34-year-old black man with acute pulmonary embolism. **Top panel:** Tracing taken in emergency room with ST-T pattern in V1 to V3 prompting admission to the CCU. **Bottom panel:** Four hours later, increased depth of T-wave inversion in V1 to V3, with now shallow T-wave inversion in leads 3 and aVF, suggested the correct diagnosis.

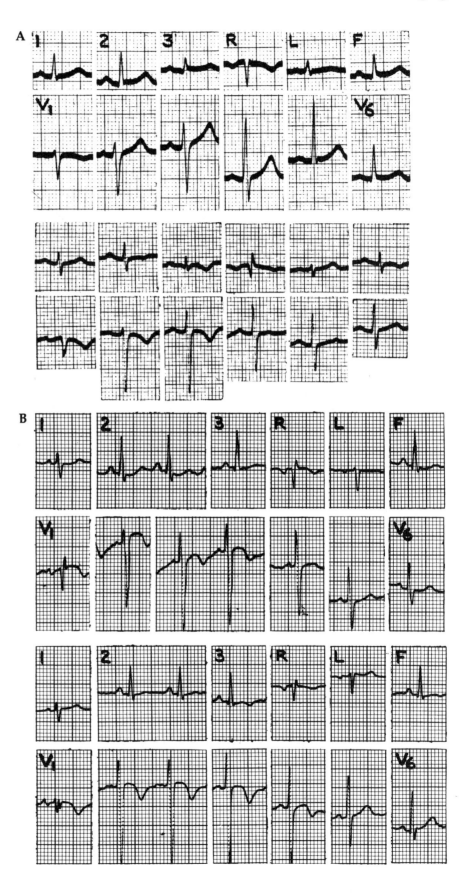

58

FIG. 58. *(continued)*

C – **Top panel:** Before pulmonary embolization. **Bottom panel:** Tracing taken on day of embolus. Note the simultaneous inversion of T3 and TV1 with no significant ST-T changes in other leads. QRS changes include development of S waves in leads 1, aVL, and V5–6, and Q wave in lead 3.

D – From a patient with massive organized embolus in the main pulmonary artery. Note the simultaneously inverted T waves in leads 3, aVF, and V1–4.

E – From a 28-year-old woman with Friedlander's pneumonia. Note the simultaneous inversion of T waves in 3, aVF, and V1-V3.

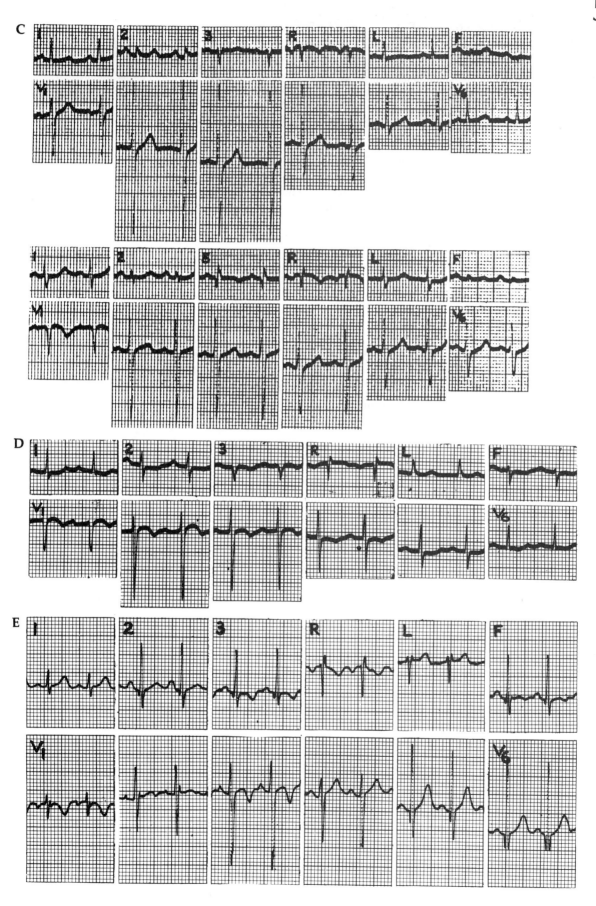

59 QS COMPLEXES IN "ANTEROSEPTAL" LEADS

Probably the most common mistake made in everyday ECG interpretation is in diagnosing anteroseptal infarction because the tracing lacks R waves in leads V1 and V2. Although this is always a possibility, a QS pattern in those two leads is more likely owing to LVH with or without incomplete LBBB, than to an anterior infarction (Fig. 59-A). A rare cause of QS complexes in "anteroseptal leads" is cardiac amyloidosis (Fig. 59-B).

A Japanese study of autopsied patients with QS complexes in any or all of leads V1 to V4 revealed the following:

IF QS COMPLEXES ARE IN	# WITH INFARCTION
V1, V2	3/15 (20%)
V1, V2, V3	6/9 (66%)
V1, V2, V3, V4	3/3 (100%)

In evaluating the significance of such QS complexes, it is important to take into account the contour of the associated ST segment and T wave. If the ST segment is concave upwards and the T wave is upright, the likely diagnosis is LVH. On the other hand, if the ST segment is convex upwards and/or the T wave is inverted, the likelihood of anteroseptal infarction greatly increases.

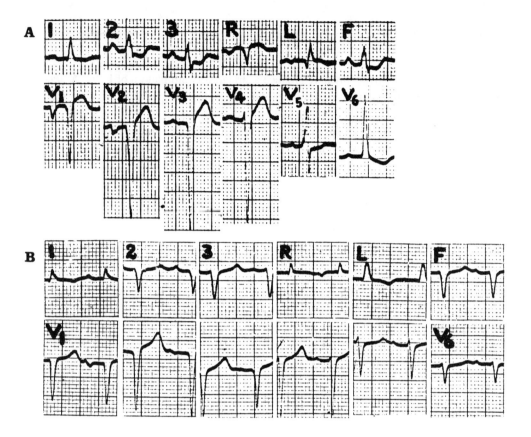

59

FIG. 59. QS COMPLEXES IN ANTEROSEPTAL LEADS

A – From a 60-year-old man with severe aortic stenosis and no sign of anteroseptal infarction at autopsy. Note the normal axis despite massive LVH.

B – From a 70-year-old man with cardiac amyloidosis.

60 HYPERTROPHIC CARDIOMYOPATHY

Hypertrophic cardiomyopathy may produce a straightforward pattern of LVH. A diagnostic sequence is an original pattern of septal hypertrophy that gradually over the years assumes the characteristics of generalized LVH.

However, a finding that is highly suggestive, but seen in only a minority of patients, is the presence of abnormal Q waves that simply do not look like the Q waves of myocardial infarction (Figs. 60-A to C).

FIG. 60. TRACINGS FROM THREE PATIENTS WITH HYPERTROPHIC CARDIOMY-OPATHY DISPLAYING Q WAVES THAT ARE CLEARLY ABNORMAL BUT UNLIKE THOSE OF MYOCARDIAL INFARCTION.

A – From a 32-year-old woman. Note the abnormal Q waves in leads 1, aVL, and V6, with tall R in V1, all indicative of septal hypertrophy.

B – Note voltage criteria for extreme LV hypertrophy, evidence of left atrial hypertrophy, with QS complexes in leads 2, 3, and aVF. (Tracing courtesy of Dr. Fred Burford.)

C – From a 29-year-old male physician. Note abnormal Q waves in leads V4-V6, as well as marked left axis deviation and impressive QRS voltage—leads V2–4 are recorded at half standard. (Reproduced from Marriott HJ. Practical Electrocardiography. 8th ed. Baltimore: Williams & Wilkins, 1988. p. 529.)

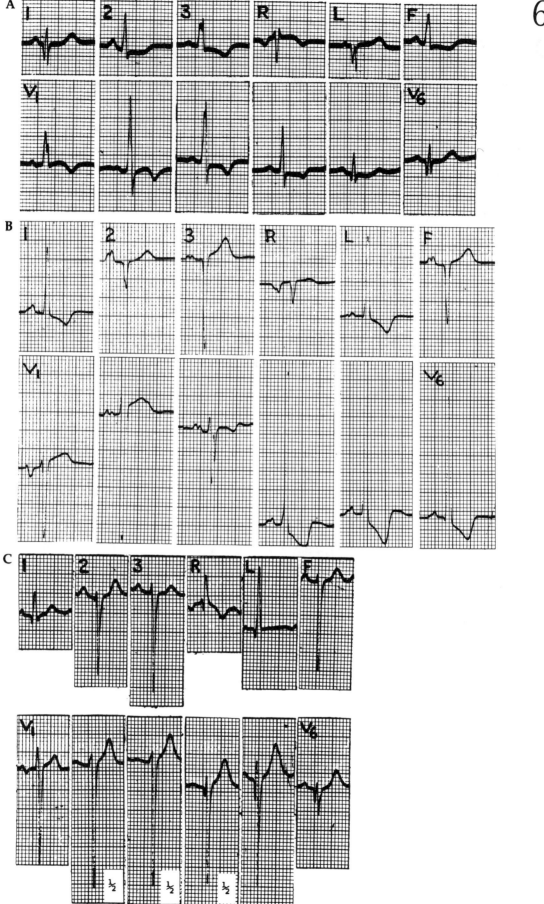

60

61 ELECTRICAL ALTERNANS

The most common cause of electrical alternans of the QRS complex is pericardial effusion (Fig. 61-A). Rarely you may find it accompanying the pulsus (mechanical) alternans of LV failure.

However, when you see total alternans, i.e., alternating amplitude not only of the QRS complexes but also of the P waves, it is virtually diagnostic of malignant pericardial effusion (Fig. 61-B).

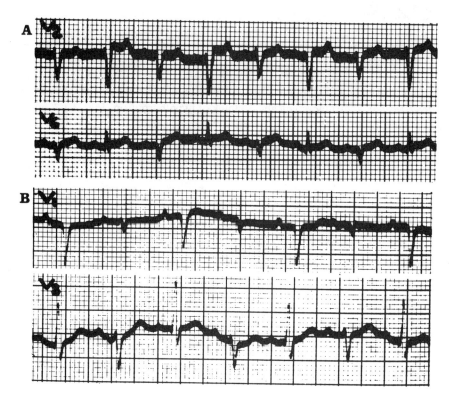

61

FIG. 61. ELECTRICAL ALTERNANS

A – From a patient having acute pericarditis with effusion.

B – "Total alternans." From a patient with malignant pericardial effusion. Note, particularly in lead V1, that the P waves as well as the QRSs alternate in amplitude.

62 HYPOTHYROIDISM

Whenever you see widespread flattening or mild inversion of T waves *without associated ST segment displacement,* always think of hypothyroidism (Figs. 62-A and C). About 50% of the time, the hunch will turn out to be correct.

The other most constant ECG finding in myxedema is low voltage of the QRS complex (Fig. 62-C). Sinus bradycardia, though often mentioned, is less often seen.

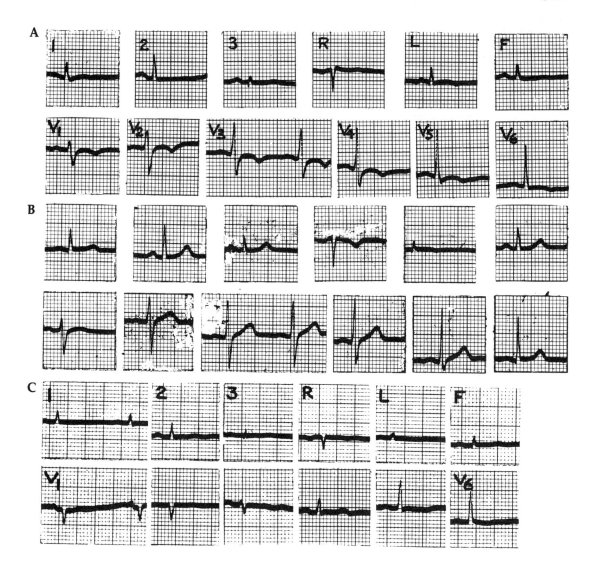

62

FIG. 62. HYPOTHYROIDISM

A – From a 38-year-old man with myxedema. Note the widespread, shallow, T-wave inversion without corresponding ST displacement.

B – Same patient after 1 month of thyroid therapy. Tracing is now entirely normal. (Tracing courtesy of Dr. Ernest Reiner.)

C – From a 45-year-old white woman with myxedema. Note the low voltage and the flat T waves without associated ST displacement.

63 CURRENTS OF INJURY

All marked ST elevations do not signal acute myocardial infarction. Acute pericarditis (Fig. 63-A), hyperkalemia (Fig. 63-B), and metastasis to the myocardium (Fig. 63-C and D) can all produce marked elevation of the ST segment (1,2). The ST elevation of pericarditis is usually unlike the other two in that the ST is concave upwards and not associated with reciprocal depression in other leads. However, it cannot be reliably differentiated from the normal variant commonly called "early repolarization" (Fig. 63-E), although the following points are helpful: 1) early repolarization is virtually a male monopoly, whereas pericarditis, of course, afflicts both sexes; 2) in early repolarization there is often a little barb at the J point that, with the ST-T, produces a "fishhook" in several leads, especially V4 and V5; and 3) in V6 the degree of ST elevation is usually less than 25 percent the height of the T wave (3). The last two clues are present in Figure 63-E.

REFERENCES

1. Hartman RB, Clark PI, Schulman P. Pronounced and prolonged ST segment elevation. A pathognomonic sign of tumor invasion of the heart. Arch Intern Med. 1982;142:1917.
2. Rosenbaum F, et al. Persistent displacement of the RS-T segment in a case of metastatic tumor of the heart. Am Heart J. 1944;27:667.
3. Spodick DH. The pericardium: a comprehensive text. Marcel Dekker Inc., NY 1997, p 59–60.

FIG. 63. EXAMPLES OF ACUTE NONINFARCTION MYOCARDIAL INJURY

A – Uremic pericarditis. Note the widespread ST elevation without reciprocal depression.

B – Hyperkalemia (K = 9.0 mEq/L) in a 3-week-old infant.

C – From a 70-year-old man with squamous cell carcinoma of the lung and metastases to the myocardium simulating acute extensive anterior infarction. (Tracing courtesy of Pamela I. Clark, R.N.; see Arch Intern Med. 1982;142:1917).

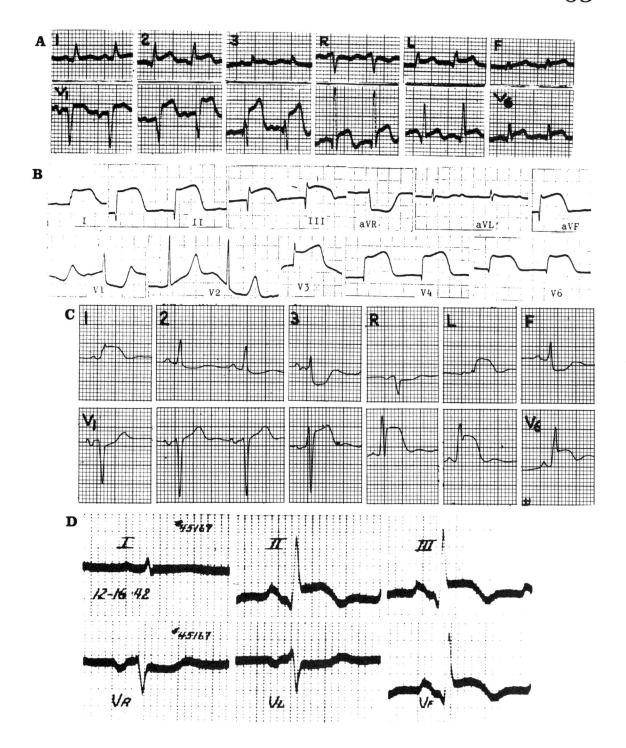

FIG. 63. *(continued)*

D – From a patient with carcinoma of the esophagus and metastases to the myocardium simulating acute inferior myocardial infarction. (Reproduced from Rosenbaum FF, et al. Am Heart J. 1944;7:667.)

63

FIG. 63. *(continued)*

E – "Early repolarization" in a 42-year old white man—not a "current of injury" but a benign variant that has to be differentiated from acute pericarditis. Note (1) the "fishhook" ST-T effect especially in leads 2, and V4–6, and (2) the T wave in V6 much taller than the level of ST elevation.

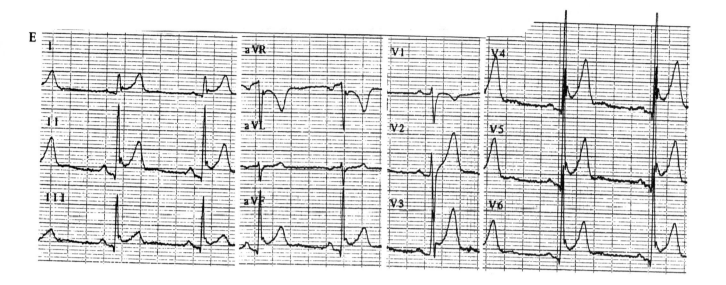

E

I   aVR   V1   V4

II   aVL   V2   V5

III   aVF   V3   V6

64 PRECORDIAL T-WAVE BALANCE

A subtle finding that is often overlooked is the TV1-taller-than-TV6 pattern (1). Although this pattern may be found in the absence of heart disease, especially when the R wave in V1 has more than usual amplitude, it should always make you look for further evidence of LV disease. For example, in the patient whose ECG is shown in Figure 64-C, it was the only herald of the infarction that was impending (Fig. 64-D).

REFERENCE

1. Weyn AS, Marriott HJ. The T-V1-taller-than-T-V6 pattern: its potential value in the early recognition of myocardial disease. Am J Cardiol. 1962;10:764.

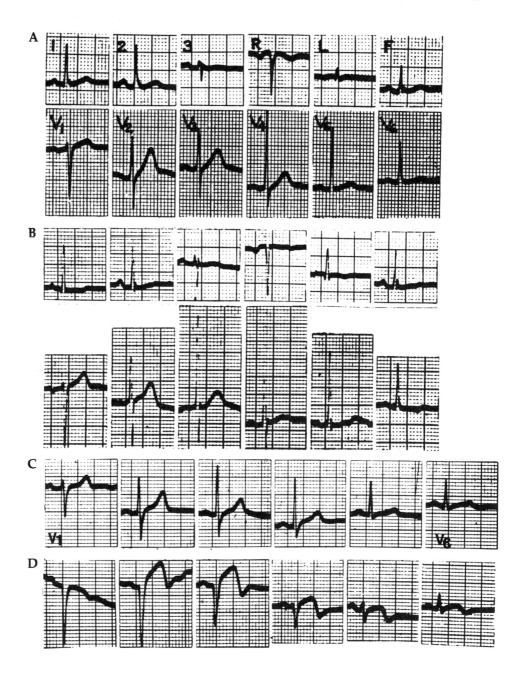

FIG. 64.

A is from a 52-year-old white man and may be reasonably considered within normal limits, although the T wave in V6 is suspiciously low and the T wave in V1 is distinctly taller. In **B,** taken 3 years later, definite ST-T abnormalities have developed in leads 1, aVL, and V6. **C** and **D** are the precordial leads (V1-V6) from a 42-year-old white-man. In **C,** the only feature of note is the T wave in V1 taller than in V6. Tracing **D,** taken 6 months after **C,** records the development of a classical anterior infarction.

65 THE OVERLOOKED U WAVE

U waves are often overlooked. In fact, some people never look for them! If you find definite inversion of the U wave in a lead where the T wave is frankly upright, it is always abnormal (Fig. 65-A). If it is found in anterior chest leads, either in a resting tracing or after exercise, it is said to be virtually diagnostic of left anterior descending coronary artery disease (1,2).

The patient whose tracing is shown in Figure 65-B was admitted on the strength of his inverted U waves (arrows) which were the only definite abnormality in his resting ECG. The next day he had typical changes of an evolving inferolateral infarction.

Inverted U waves may be the main or only abnormal finding in an exercise test (Fig. 65-C), or the sole residuum in the wake of a variant anginal attack (Fig. 65-D).

REFERENCES

1. Gerson MC, McHenry PL. Resting U wave inversion as a marker of stenosis of the left anterior descending coronary artery. Am J Med. 1980;69:545.
2. Gerson MC, et al. Exercise-induced U-wave inversion as a marker of stenosis of the left anterior descending coronary artery. Circulation. 1979;60:1014.

FIG. 65

A – Note the subtle inversion of U waves (arrow).

B – From a 77-year-old surgeon with chest discomfort whose ECG next day showed acute inferolateral infarction. Note the subtle inversion of U waves in leads V2-V5 (arrows).

C – Lead V4 recorded before and after exercise in a 38-year-old man with chest pain. The most striking positive feature of the post-exercise tracing is gross U wave inversion (arrow). (Reproduced from Marriott HJ. Practical Electrocardiography. 8th ed. Baltimore: Williams & Wilkins, 1988, p. 460.)

D – Tracing recorded during an attack of variant angina—the figures indicate time elapsed since onset of pain. Note that at 8′ 15″ (bottom strip), the tracing has returned to normal except for monumental U wave inversion (arrows).

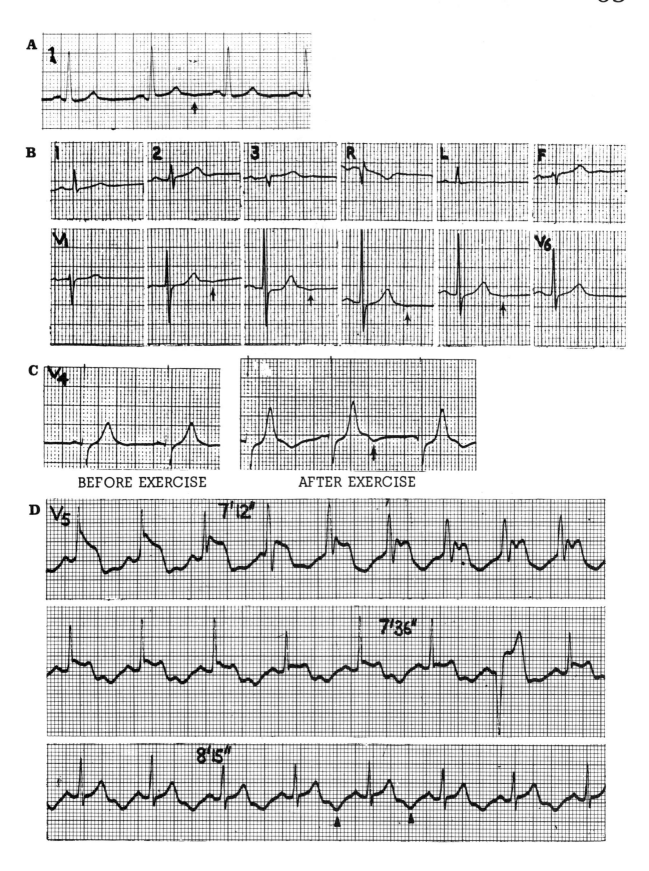

65

A

B

C

BEFORE EXERCISE   AFTER EXERCISE

D

66 HYPOKALEMIA AND ITS MIMIC

Potassium depletion produces characteristic changes in the ECG. Fluctuations in intracellular concentration of potassium produce a seesaw effect between the T wave and the U wave—as the T wave becomes lower the U wave gets taller, and vice versa. At a level of about 2.7 meq/L, T and U waves are usually of approximately equal height (Fig. 66-A). If the concentration decreases further, the ST segment becomes mildly depressed, the U wave towers over the T wave and, in fact, there is often no clear-cut dividing line between them so that the ST-T-U amalgam produces a long, drawn-out roller-coaster effect (Fig. 66-B). Some liken the resulting curves to a flattened "S" lying on its side. It is this long, drawn-out double curve, without visible separation of T from U wave, that has led to the mistaken belief that the QT interval is lengthened by hypokalemia. When hypokalemia produces the "camel-hump" T-U effect and makes it clear where the T wave ends (as in leads V2 and V3 of Fig. 66-A), it becomes evident that the Q-T interval is not prolonged.

The summation of digitalis and quinidine effects can produce an indistinguishable ST-T-U pattern. Quinidine provides the prominent U wave, while digitalis lowers the T wave and depresses the ST segment. Figures 66-C and D compare and contrast the pattern of hypokalemia with that of the combined drug effects.

FIG. 66.

A to C – Three classic patterns of hypokalemia. In **A,** K+ = 2.8 meq/L. Note the camel-hump pattern in V2 and V3 with T and U waves of approximately equal height.

In **B,** K+ = 1.5 mEq/L. Note that there is ST depression and the U wave now towers over the T wave.

In **C,** K+ = 2.3 mEq/L. Note how well this pattern of hypokalemia is imitated by combined drug effects of digitalis and quinidine (see **D**).

D – Combined digitalis and quinidine effects in an 85-year-old man with congestive heart failure whose K+ was 4.0 mEq/L.

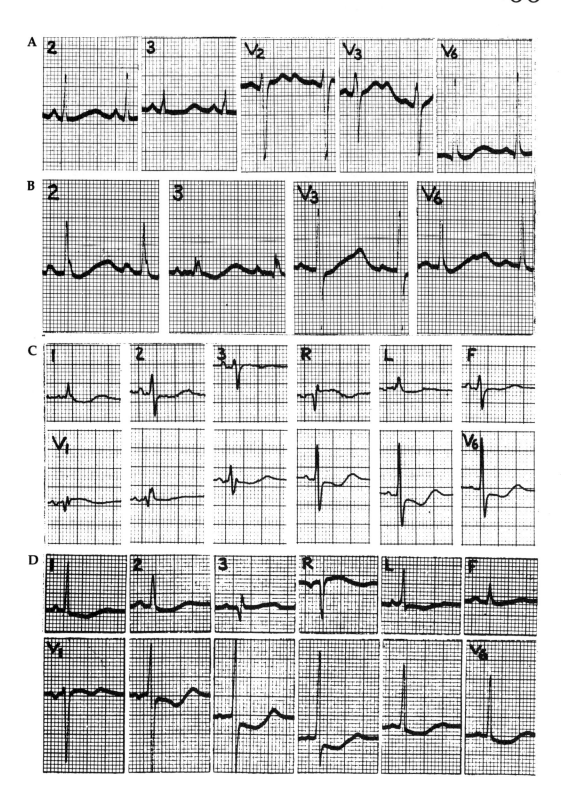

66

67 THE ISOELECTRIC BIPOLAR LEAD

A common blunder-cum-deception is the reversal or otherwise misplacement of the limb electrodes of bipolar leads. Many a bizarre pattern can result from such misplacements.

One form of misplacement is easy to spot, yet often goes unrecognized. If both electrodes for one of the bipolar limb leads wind up on the two legs, that lead will have practically nothing to say for itself, because there is virtually no potential difference between the two legs as far as the heart is concerned. The tracing of that supposed bipolar lead is therefore almost a straight line (lead 1 in Figs. 67-A and B, and lead 3 in Figs. 67-C and D). With the two arm electrodes for lead 1 on the two legs (Figs. 67-A and B), naturally the leg electrodes must be on the arms. So leads 2, 3, and aVF will be upside down simulating inferior infarction as in Figure 67-A. And the aVR and aVL leads will look virtually identical since each of them is on one leg. If the two electrodes of lead 3 (left arm and left leg) find themselves on the two legs (Figs. 67-C and D), leads 1 and 2 will be virtually identical, and so will leads aVL and aVF.

FIG. 67.

A – This tracing was originally interpreted as acute inferior infarction because of the Q waves, ST elevation, and T-wave inversion in leads 2, 3, and aVF. The missed tip-off was the almost straight line in lead 1 suggesting that the two electrodes for this lead were attached to the two legs. The bottom panel presents the patient's limb leads correctly attached.

B – Ventricular tachycardia with arm electrodes on legs.

C – In this case with acute inferior infarction, the left arm electrode is attached to the right leg. Here the tip-off is the almost straight line in lead 3 (plus, of course, the unusual distribution of ST elevation).

D – Normal ECG with left arm and right leg electrodes reversed so that both electrodes for lead 3 are on the legs.

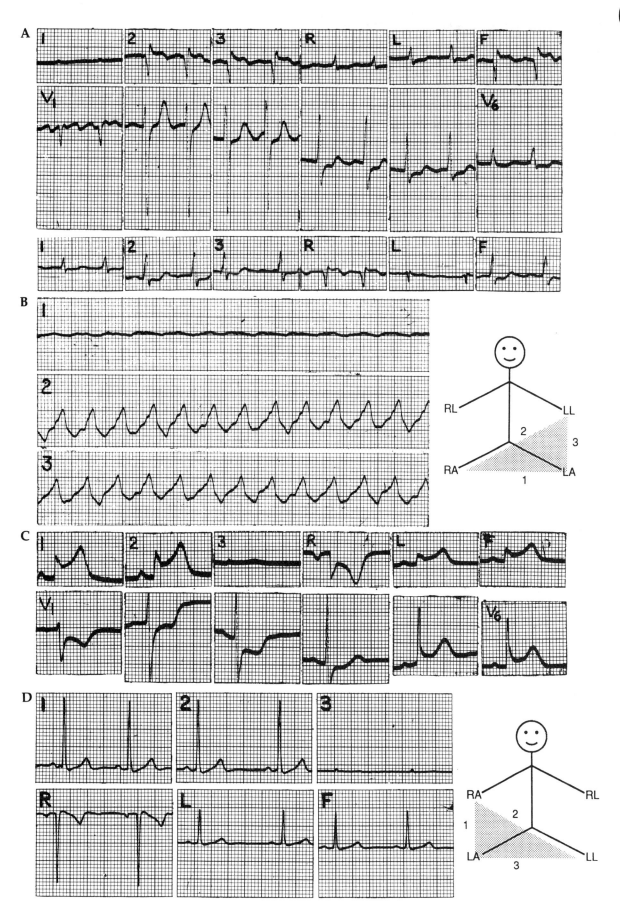

67

68 THE BIPOLAR EQUATION

Einthoven's equation states that lead 2 = lead 1 + lead 3—in other words, the waves and complexes in leads 1 and 3 together add up algebraically to the corresponding waves and complexes in lead 2. A knowledge of this equation can explain some otherwise apparent inconsistencies. In Figure 68-A, the sinus P waves in leads 2 and 3 are so similar that no P wave is visible in lead 1—it's there, but it's flat and invisible!—and from that lead alone, surely most observers would diagnose junctional rhythm.

Both Figures 68-B and C are examples of RBBB in which the QRS in one of the limb leads looks normally narrow: lead 2 in Figure 68-B and lead 1 in Figure 68-C. In Figure 68-B the negative S wave in lead 1 counterbalances the terminal part of the positive R in lead 3 so that, by Einthoven's equation, nothing is left over for lead 2 and the terminal part of the QRS is therefore isoelectric in that lead. In Figure 68-C, the terminal negative waves in leads 2 and 3 are equal, therefore there is nothing left over for lead 1 and the terminal part of the QRS is isoelectric in that lead.

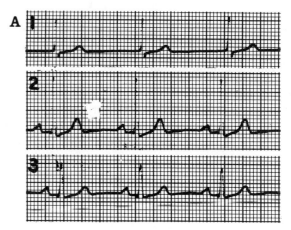

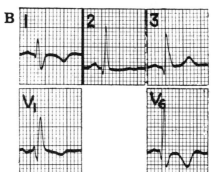

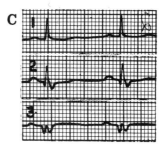

68

69 BEWARE THE FREEZE

One of the hazards of modern monitoring is misdiagnosis resulting from artifacts produced by the ability to freeze and then record without a telltale marker to indicate that the trace was frozen. Figure 69 presents a selection of artifacts deliberately produced by freezing and unfreezing the tracing at strategic moments. Thus one can simulate sinus node reentry, shortening or lengthening of the P-R interval, the momentary development of bundle branch block, and pairing of ventricular extrasystoles. Such artifacts can be produced inadvertently and then be innocently included in the patient's record.

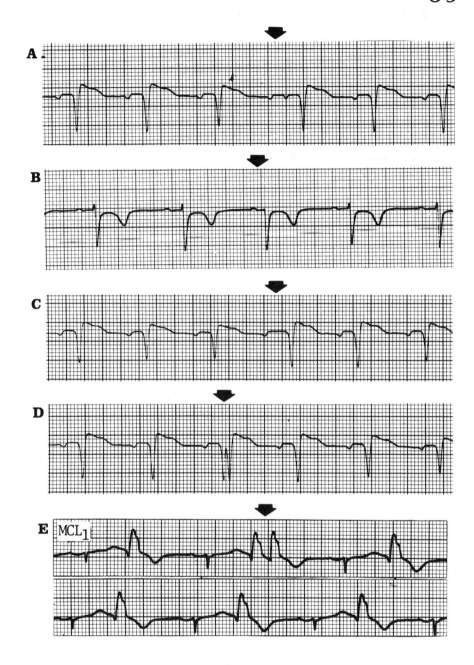

69

FIG. 69. ARTIFACTS PRODUCED BY FREEZING AND THAWING THE MONITORING TRACE

Simulations of:

A – Sinus node reentry.

B – Shortening of P-R interval.

C – First degree A-V block.

D – Intermittent BBB.

E – Paired ventricular extrasystoles.

70 REPOLARIZATION ALTERNANS

Alternation of the T and/or U wave without accompanying QRS alternation is an intriguing, unexplained phenomenon that has been described in—among other conditions—LV failure, hypochloremic alkalosis with hypokalemia, hypocalcemia, hypomagnesemia, head trauma, and the Romano-Ward syndrome following ventricular fibrillation. It seems particularly to affect patients in extremis following resuscitative efforts.

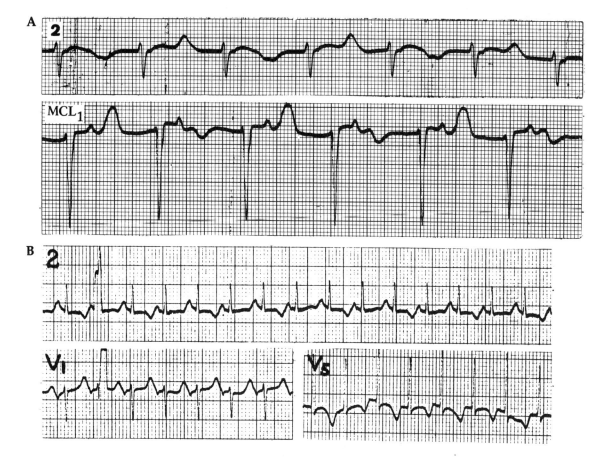

70

FIG. 70

A – Alternation of T and U waves without QRS alternans. From a 64-year-old black man with hypertension, hyperkalemia, hypocalcemia, respiratory arrest, ventricular fibrillation, and seizures.

B – From a 5-week-old baby girl with acute myocarditis precipitating cardiac arrest. Repolarization alternans recorded following resuscitation. (Tracing courtesy of Dr. Hughes Day.)

INDEX

All initial entries are nouns. Italic page numbers indicate figures. Page numbers followed by the letter t indicate tables.

Keep Your Assessment Skills At Their Peak.

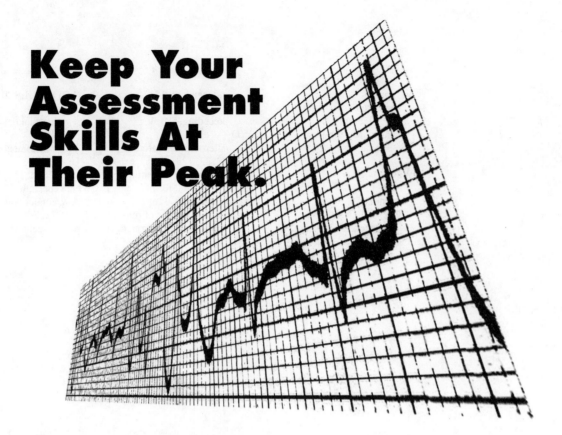

Rhythm Quizlets
Self Assessment

Second Edition

Henry J. L. Marriott, MD

Arrhythmias are masters of disguise. That's why **Rhythm Quizlets, Second Edition** covers all the variations you'll encounter in the electrocardiogram—from simple extrasystole and the uncomplicated Wenckebach period to the concealed junctional extrasystole and concealed super normal conduction.

Renowned diagnostician Dr. Henry Marriott divides the book into three "zones" based on difficulty. Whether you want to learn to recognize arrhythmias or sharpen your diagnostic skills, there's an appropriate comfort area. You can enter:

- **The Green Zone**: An excellent introduction to straightforward disturbances for beginners.
- **The Yellow Zone**: It's more treacherous, with potholes and detours that complicate diagnosis.
- **The Red Zone:** Deserves a huge caution flag. It's loaded with pitfalls and booby traps, with a number of complicated tracings that demand optimum skill and expertise.

The second edition is updated with 75 new tracings, more than half covering the recent advances in the three-lead format.

Get in the zone with Dr. Marriott. You'll never look at arrhythmias the same way again.

We invite you to preview this text for a full month. If you're not completely satisfied, return it at no further obligation (US and Canada only).

Phone orders accepted 24 hours a day, 7 days a week (US only). Prices subject to change without notice.

From the US:
Call: 1-800-638-0672
Fax: 1-800-447-8438

From Canada:
Call: 1-800-665-1148
Fax: 1-800-665-0103

From outside the US and Canada:
Call: 410-528-4223
Fax: 410-528-8550

VISIT US ON THE INTERNET!
E-mail: custserv@wwilkins.com
Home page: http://www.wwilkins.com

MARBCCBIA   97
→ S7B453